The

«ASCS»

Inpatient Admission Scheduling and Control System

WALTON M. HANCOCK

PAUL F. WALTER

AUPHA Press
Ann Arbor, Michigan
Washington, D.C.

1983

Library of Congress Cataloging in Publication Data

Hancock, Walton M., 1929-
    The "ASCS" : inpatient scheduling and control
system.

    Bibliography: p.
    1. ASCS (Computer system) 2. Hospitals--Admission
and discharge. 3. Medical appointments and schedules.
4. Hospital utilization. I. Walter, Paul F.,
1948-   . II. Title. III. Title: "A.S.C.S."
[DNLM: 1. Appointments and schedules. 2. Automatic
data processing. 3. Hospital administration.
4. Patient care planning. 5. Patient admission.
WX 162 H235a]
RA971.8.H36 1983   362.1'1'0685   83-11789
ISBN 0-914904-92-2

AUPHA Press is an imprint of Health Administration Press.

Health Administration Press   Association of University Programs
School of Public Health   in Health Administration
The University of Michigan   1911 North Fort Myer Drive, Suite 503
Ann Arbor, Michigan 48109   Arlington, Virginia 22209
(313) 764-1380   (703) 524-5500

TABLE OF CONTENTS

PREFACE

The "ASCS" - Inpatient Admissions Scheduling and Control System was written to provide the hospital administrator, the Director of Admissions, the management engineer and the hospital planner with a better understanding of the potential of computer-aided technology to obtain superior use of the beds of hospitals.

Chapters I, II, III and VI have been written for the individual who wants to obtain a general understanding of the admissions process and what has been accomplished using the ASCS. Chapters IV and VIII are for those interested in maintaining the ASCS after it is operating. Chapter V contains information useful to hospital planners, administrators and management engineers who want to determine the number of beds or the occupancies that can be achieved using the ASCS. Chapter VII contains a description of the patient flow information necessary to develop the admission decision rules. Future extensions of the ASCS for operating room scheduling and the more appropriate staffing of services is contained in Chapter IX.

The authors wish to thank George Gamota, Director of the Institute of Science and Technology, for his assistance in obtaining support, Marietha Forester and Jan Eckert for their typing and organizational assistance, and Roger Guiles and David Peelle for editing the manuscript.

Walton M. Hancock
Paul F. Walter
June 1983

CHAPTER I

INTRODUCTION

A.   The Philosophy of the ASCS

The ASCS, an acronym for the Admission Scheduling and
Control System, is a philosophy, a methodology, and a system
designed to accomplish the acts of admitting inpatients to a
hospital. As a philosophy, its design objectives require it to
be responsive to and achieve its host hospital's specific
policies concerning occupancies, patient placement, numbers of
patients scheduled, and provisions for emergency admissions. At
the same time, the philosophy requires the system to provide an
environment conducive to the delivery of quality care. As a
system, it places overall responsibility and control of the
admissions process in the hands of the hospital administration.
As a methodology, day-to-day decisions are carried out by the
hospital's admissions office. This is as it should be.

Unlike many systems, the ASCS is sufficiently flexible so
that its specific design objectives are determined by the
individual hospital rather than having them "forced" upon the
hospital by the system. The ASCS can be implemented in community
hospitals with only a few major clinical services as well as in
large teaching hospitals where the need exists to be responsive
to a number of clinical services and subspecialties. Intensive
care units, coronary care units and progressive (step-down) care
units may be designed into the system according to their function
established by hospital policy. Where appropriate, the holding
area resources of emergency room facilities can also be included
in overall system design.

Typical of frequently selected major ASCS objectives is to
"Maximize inpatient occupancies subject to: 1) keeping surgical
cancellations due to lack of beds to less than an average of two
per month and 2) to keeping situations where there is not a
licensed bed for emergency arrivals to less than an average of
two per month." With this objective in mind, a cost control role
is performed through realizing maximum use of the facility.
Concurrently, by controlling occupancy levels and rates of
admission, the occurrence of adverse situations at high frequency
levels is avoided (i.e., surgical cancellations, hereafter called
cancellations; and no licensed beds for emergency patients,
hereafter called emergency turnaways). Combined with additional
stipulations providing for average minimum unit occupancies,
minimum average rates of admission to particular clinical
services, etc., the objectives reflect the basic system
philosophy of promoting the most appropriate use of the
hospital's resources in a quality care context.

High average occupancies and greatly reduced problems with
cancellations and turnaways are the main benefits that have been
realized from the ASCS system. Also, the ASCS provides for

other potential benefits that have yet to be fully explored. A number have been pursued to the point of clearly establishing their potential. These are as follows:

1. Higher average unit and hospital-wide occupancies tend to stabilize the workload of many hospital personnel, particularly those in nursing and in the ancillary service departments. More stable loads make scheduling and the determination of the appropriate numbers of personnel easier (1 & 2). Assuming that stabilized occupancies result in more stable workloads and personnel schedules, a reduction in staff tensions may also be inferred.

2. Scheduling beds at the same time as surgery increases the potential for stabilizing the workload for the operating room staff and therefore increasing the potential to get much higher utilization from the operating rooms. In many cases, overtime and staff costs can be sharply reduced (3).

3. The potential for reducing length of stay through pre-admissions testing is enhanced because of the ability to advance schedule larger numbers of patient admissions (4).

4. The potential exists to reduce the number of emergency patient admissions. In many non-ASCS hospitals, patients are admitted as emergencies that are really only urgent in nature (need to be admitted within the next few days but not immediately). As we shall see later, part of this is due to the hospital's use of the typical admission system that literally forces medicine service physicians to declare patients as emergency in order to get them admitted. With an ASCS urgent admissions process, physicians do not have to resort to declaring patients emergency in order to get them admitted. As a result, hospital emergency admissions are reduced, thus enabling average occupancies to be increased and reducing the chances of having to cancel surgery (4).

5. Allocations of beds among services can be more equitably accomplished. Based on the same historical analysis of patient flows used for ASCS implementation, determinations of how many beds should be allocated to each service are routinely made. Considerations for bed allocations are of particular importance in large teaching hospitals because of the competition for beds between a large number of clinical services (See Chapter V for references).

6. Superior planning for additional facilities can be made and with greater precision than with contemporary methods. The ASCS Simulator has been used to construct bed-sizing algorithms. These algorithms can be used to determine, with stated precision, the number of beds to be used given a patient population to be served or the occupancy that can be achieved for a given number of beds (5, 6 & 7).

The original version of ASCS was developed at the University of Michigan under a grant from the National Center for Health Services Research, Resources Administration; Department of HEW, Health PHS Grant no. HS 00228, and a W.K. Kellogg Foundation Grant. The results of this work are reported in various publications (8, 9, 10, 11, 12, 13, 14, 15), the most widely distributed being a book, "Cost Control in Hospitals"(4). The system has been installed in a number of hospitals by staff members of the University of Michigan, the Greater Detroit Area Hospital Council, O.R., Inc. and by Walton M. Hancock Inc.

B. Implementation of the ASCS

Briefly, the process of implementation of the ASCS is as follows:

1. Specific hospital objectives for the ASCS are determined by discussions with hospital administration.

2. Data are collected, usually from a medical record abstracting process, consisting of: types, numbers of patients, services to which the patients were admitted and transferred on the respective days of their length of stay. At least six months of data are required with twelve months being preferred. If the data presently available are determined to be inadequate, then the establishment of a reasonable data collection methodology must be implemented as soon as possible.

3. Initially the data are used to determine length of stay distributions and arrival and transfer rates for each of the clinical services. The emphasis of this analysis is to produce a model that accurately describes the admission and patient flow processes during the period covered by the data collection.

4. The data in step 3 are then used as input to the ASCS Simulator to determine the decision rules needed to satisfy the specific system objectives of step 1. These decision rules, when implemented, will direct admissions office personnel in their day-to-day decisions regarding occupancies, number of elective patients to schedule, urgent admission policies, and the provisions for emergency patients.

5. The admissions department personnel and the operating room personnel are taught the decision rules and the rationales behind them.

6. System control charts are established to ensure that system objectives are being met and to enable management to change the decision rules as the patient mix changes.

7. A system starting date is determined at which time the decision rules are used on-line by admissions office personnel.

8. Someone in the hospital, usually from Management Engineering, is taught to change the decision rules using the simulator so that the system can be maintained and/or changed to reflect hospital policies as they change (Chapter VII contains the detailed instructions on how to do this).

C.   The Relation of the ASCS to the Budget

Hospitals are labor-intensive organizations for which the budget represents the plan for the resources to be used by the patients admitted to the hospital. The budget, usually implicitly and in a macrosense, is based on the assumption that a certain number of patients with a certain mix of needs will be admitted during the budget horizon. Thus every time a patient is admitted to the hospital, a certain amount of the hospital's resources are committed. Since a labor-intensive organization is involved, the majority of budgeted resources (labor) that is available (budgeted) but not needed by the patients is a sunk cost; i.e., it is paid for but no benefit is received.

To budget sufficient resources to care for the patients with no excess would be ideal. This, however, is probably impossible to achieve, but it is important to get as close to this goal as possible. Thus a system that provides control over admissions should enable the hospital over time to budget with minimum sunk costs. Increases in maximum average occupancies, stabilization of the workloads of nurses and ancillary personnel and the potential for improved operating room scheduling are examples of the potentials for better planning (budgeting) through the analysis and control of patient admissions. Chapter V contains examples of the economic potential of closely matching consumption with budgeted resources (patient admissions with budgets).

D.   A Summary of the Results Achieved

The ASCS was originally implemented in Baker Hospital in 1976 (4). To date there have been a number of implementations yielding sufficient data to demonstrate the results achieved. The results, of course, are a function of the objectives that the hospital was (is) attempting to accomplish. They are presented in three categories: dollar savings, reductions in internal tensions (reduced cancellations and turnaways), and improvements in the planning process.

1. Dollar Reductions

Figure I-1 is a summary of the dollar savings as reported in the literature. The authors have also been involved with several other institutions; the estimated savings are summarized in Figure I-2.

HOSPITAL	DOCUMENTATION REFERENCE	DOCUMENTED SAVINGS	IMPLEMENTATION COST
Baker Hospital	4	$530,000/yr.	$30,000
Greater S.E. Community Hospital	16	$750,000/yr.	$30,000
Botsford General Hospital	17	Approx. $426,000/3 yrs.	$25,000
Wyandotte General Hospital	17	$131,400/3 yrs.	Unknown
St. Thomas Hospital	18	$144,400/yr.	$25,000

Figure I-1.* The Savings and Installation Costs of the Implementation of the ASCS System

Hospital	Savings & Costs
x	A predicted increase in revenues of $10,000,000/yr. due to an increase in occupancy. Cost of installation: $60,000.
y	A predicted savings of $1,800,000/yr. due to increasing occupancy 4.2%. Cost of installation: $51,000.
z	Reduction of 20 beds due to raising occupancy. Cost of installation: $45,000.

Figure I-2. More Data of Less Precise Nature Concerning Dollar Savings

*Figures I-1 and I-3 are reproduced with permission from: Proceedings from "Inpatient Admissions Systems", Hancock, Walton M., 10th IMACS World Congress on System Simulation & Scientific Computation, Montreal, Canada, 08/82, pp. 213-215

In all cases, the savings have greatly exceeded the cost of installation.

2. Reductions in Internal Tensions

Reductions in internal tensions occur when there are reductions in the numbers of turnaways and/or cancellations. Figure I-3 is a summary of the data available concerning surgical cancellations and turnaways prior to and following system implementation.

Hospital	Reference	Cancellations and Turnaways Prior to ASCS		Cancellations and Turnaways With ASCS	
		Surgery Can./MTH	Emergency Turn./MTH	Surgery Can./MTH	Emergency Turn./MTH
BAKER	4	10	(4)	1	(4)
DELTA	10	49	0	1 (2)***	0 (2)
x	–	52	0*	8 (8)	8** (8)
CHARLES	8	18	–	9 (6)	0 (2)
z	–	27	0*	4 (4)	4** (4)

     *   Rerouting of emergency patients to another hospital
          frequently occurred.
   **   Assuming no rerouting of emergency patients to
          another hospital.
 *** The numbers in parentheses were part of the system
          design objectives.

Figure I-3. A Summary of the Changes in Surgery Cancellation and Emergency Turnaways with ASCS Implementation

The results are that turnaways and cancellations were sharply reduced by ASCS and that, with rare exceptions, the design objectives were met or exceeded.

3. Improvements in the Planning Process

The ASCS simulator has been used in several ways to aid in the planning of how many beds are needed and to what service they should be allocated. The following is a brief list of applications.

      a. New Hospitals--The Management Information Systems
         Group of the Department of Hospital Administration at
         the University of Michigan contracted with the
         University of Michigan Hospital to aid in the

determination of the number of beds needed for its new facility (7). Further, the simulator was used to help determine the effects on the ancillary services due to the scheduling of both inpatients and outpatients (1).

    b. The Simulator was used to determine the occupancy at which a large pediatric hospital could operate and still have the patients treated according to existing policy (5).

    c. In at least one-half of the ASCS implementations, questions have arisen and been answered concerning the appropriate sizes of the units so that transfers between units can be reduced. These questions have been so frequent that special bed sizing algorithms were developed and are covered in Chapter V of this book.

E. Perceptions by the Users

The ASCS was purposely designed so that, in general, all of the powerful actors, both administrators and physicians, would benefit by the system. However, what is perceived as a benefit is in the eyes of the beholder and what may be a benefit to one group may be of no consequence to another. The following are typical:

1. The Administration

    a. The previous section gives a summary of the money saved -- either by the hospital or by the community. Providing the necessary services at reduced costs is an administrative responsibility to which many hospital administrators are becoming increasingly sensitive. Thus prior to implementation, the expected savings (or potential increases in revenue) are computed and compared to the cost of implementation. Typical rates of return have been given in the previous section.

    b. High numbers of surgical cancellations and the need to use hall beds for emergency patients cause a great deal of inconvenience for the patients, medical staffs involved and result in conflicts with administration. By keeping the number of surgical cancellations and the need for hall beds (or emergency turnaways) to acceptable levels (which have been negotiated between administrative and hospital staffs in advance), tensions are greatly reduced, thus enabling administration to devote its time to other more constructive tasks.

2. The Surgeons

   a. The surgeons' first concern when presented with the details of the ASCS system is that they are going to be restricted as to when they can do surgery. This is partly true. No longer are they going to be able to get surgery posted without the O.R. posting people having to follow the hospital policy as embedded in the decision rules regarding bed availability. However, surgical cancellations will be sharply reduced if they were high prior to ASCS. In addition, they can do at least as much surgery as they have in the past and potentially more because the ASCS enables the hospital to be run at higher maximum average occupancies.

   b. The elective surgery schedules established so that they are very close to the average rates of admission prior to implementation for each day of the week. This fact in general enables the surgeons to operate on the same days before and after implementation.

   c. The surgeons are able to get firm dates for hospital admission when they schedule O.R. time. These are guaranteed by the hospital with a very high probability -- usually 99 out of a 100.

3. Physicians Other Than Surgeons

   a. The typical hospital admissions system, which is discussed in Chapter II, gives the non-surgeons the available beds after elective surgical patients are admitted. This process frequently forces the non-surgeon physicians to declare patients emergent in order to get them admitted. If the hospital has an urgent admissions category, the policies regarding admission within a specified number of days are usually not followed, causing the non-surgeons to react by declaring their urgent patients emergent. The ASCS system stabilizes surgical admissions, thus enabling an urgent admission system to function. Policies concerning required admission of urgent patients within a specified number of days are frequently instituted and enforced. Thus the non-surgeons have what they perceive to be a more organized and rational method of getting their patients admitted.

   b. Medical service physicians increasingly need to schedule patients for special procedures. Thus there is a demand to have scheduled medical patients as well as scheduled surgical patients. Where this need exists, the ASCS can provide the necessary decision rules.

4. Admissions Office Personnel

The ASCS is designed to provide the admissions office with decision rules that enable them to carry out hospital policy. But, the system is also designed to encourage the admissions office to take initiatives to increase the effectiveness of the system's decision rules by (1) instituting systems to encourage discharge if it is perceived that surgical cancellations are likely to occur, (2) keeping administration informed of changes in patient mix and physician practice and (3) more fully integrating their activities with the O.R. posting personnel.

The reaction of admissions personnel to the system has been favorable, probably because they feel that they have better control of the situation. If there is a problem and they have followed the decision rules, the system is at fault, not them. The system also enables the admissions personnel to effectively resist pressures by individual physicians to admit patients if the admission is contrary to policy. The admissions personnel are not expected to "take the heat" themselves, but to refer the physician to the proper administrative or medical official.

5. Operating Room Personnel

In most cases, prior to ASCS, the O.R. posting personnel did not have to worry about bed availability. When scheduling elective surgical procedures, with ASCS, the daily limits of admissions for elective surgical procedures also have to be taken into account. The O.R. posting personnel have no difficulty doing this, but in the early stages of implementation, they receive pressure from surgeons. Once they realize that they can refer surgeons to their Chief of the service or to the administration, they feel much better about the system. Also, the pressure from the surgeons exists for only the first few weeks of implementation and is therefore of short duration.

6. The Patients

Although no poll has been taken of patients, physicians have told the authors that their patients react very favorably to firm dates of admission and to positive statements by the admissions office personnel regarding their admission status. Even when the patient is on the urgent waiting list, the admissions people can make reasonably good estimates of when the patient will be admitted. The system does reduce the uncertainty of when admission will occur and thus is perceived favorably by patients. The favorable response by patients also causes the physicians to be more supportive.

F. References

1. Hancock, W. and Walter, P. "University Hospital Ancillary Services Project." Report 80-1, Bureau of Hospital Administration, January 1980.

2. Hancock, W. and Fuhs, P. "The Effect of The Budgeting Process on Nurse Staffing," (Report 82-1, Bureau of Hospital Administration, Feb. 1982.

3. Magerlein, J. "Surgical Scheduling and Admissions Control," Report No. 78-6, Bureau of Hospital Administration, University of Michigan, Nov. 1978 (Ph.D. Thesis).

4. Cost Control in Hospitals, edited by W. Hancock, J. Griffith, and F. Munson, Health Administration Press, The University of Michigan, Ann Arbor, Michigan, 1976.

5. Hancock, A.; Magerlein, D.; Hancock, W.; and Walter, P. "A Case Example of the Determination of Maximum Average Occupancy of a 215-Bed Pediatric Hospital," Bureau of Hospital Administration, The University of Michigan, Report No. 79-4, March 1979.

6. Goodall, W.; Hancock, W.; Walter, P.; Macy, B.; Storer, R.; and Buttrey, S. "Cost Savings Analysis Using Hospital Activity Measures," Bureau of Hospital Administration, University of Michigan, Report #76-2, Dec. 1976.

7. Hancock, W.; Johnston, C.; Magerlein, D.; Martin, J.; and Walter, P. "Replacement Hospital Bed Size: Determination and Final Results," Bureau of Hospital Administration, University of Michigan, Report No. 78-1, May 1978.

8. Yannitelli, P. and Hancock, W. "Implementation of the ASCS into Charles Hospital," Report 75-3, Bureau of Hospital Administration, The University of Michigan, June, 1975.

9. Yannitelli, P.; Hancock, W.; and Fleming, J. "The Development of a Scheduling System for a Surgical Wing of El Camino Hospital, " Report 74-3, Bureau of Hospital Administration, The University of Michigan, November, 1974.

10. Johnston, C.; Hancock, W.; and Steiger, D. "The First Three Months of Implementation of the Admission Scheduling and Control System at Delta Hospital," Ann Arbor, Michigan: Bureau of Hospital Administration, The University of Michigan, Report No. 75-9, November 1975.

11. Walter, P. and Hancock, W. "The Admission Scheduling and
     Control System: A Comprehensive Hospital Admissions
     Modeling and Simulation System II," Report 77-1, Bureau of
     Hospital Administration, The University of Michigan, May,
     1977.

12. Hancock, W.; Warner, D.; Heda, S.; and Fuhs, P. "Admissions
     Scheduling and Control System," Report 74-2, Bureau of
     Hospital Administration, September 1974.

13. Hancock, W.; Hamilton, R.; and Hawley, K. "The Admissions
     Scheduling and Control System: The Admissions Simulator",
     Bureau of Hospital Administration, The University of
     Michigan, Report No. 75-1, February 1975.

14. Hancock, W.; Magerlein, D.; Storer, R.; and Martin, J.
     "Parameters Affecting Hospital Occupancy and Implications
     for Facility Sizing, "Health Services Research, Fall,
     1978.

15. Hancock, W.; Martin, J.; and Storer, R. "Simulation-Based
     Occupancy Recommendations for Adult Medical/Surgical Units
     Using Admissions Scheduling System," Inquiry, Vol. XV, No.
     1, pp. 25-32.

16. "Reducing Hospital Costs," Washington Post, 18 July 1977,
     p.1.

17. "Management Improvement to Reduce Costs Project (MIRC)," M.
     Needleman, L. Fahle, D. Seiger, J. Miller and F. Butler,
     Greater Detroit Area Hospital Council, Inc., October,
     1977.

18. Day, E. "The Development and Implementation of a Patient
     Scheduling and Control System," Clearinghouse for Hospital
     Management Engineering, Proceedings of a Forum, April
     24-25, 1980, Portland, Oregon.

CHAPTER II

EXAMPLES OF TYPICAL HOSPITAL ADMISSIONS SYSTEMS

A.   Introduction

For purposes of comparison, examples of typical hospital admission systems are presented. These systems are of two types: those used in community hospitals and those used by teaching/tertiary hospitals. Since the teaching/tertiary hospital admissions system is a modification of the system originally developed for community hospitals, the community hospital system will be presented first.

B.   The "Evolved" Community Hospital System

The admissions process in the typical community hospital is what is known in systems technology as an "evolved" system. As such, it is a system that has been "put together" by admissions personnel over many years to meet the perceived objectives of the institution. The basics of the system are as follows:

1. Excess Operating Room Capacity

Most hospitals have an excess of O.R. capacity. The typical O.R. utilization is between 45% and 63% of the available staff time (1, 2). On any given day the number of operations that are scheduled by operating room personnel, whose responsibility is to make sure that there is sufficient O.R. time available on the day of the procedure, will vary widely. Once the patient is scheduled in the O.R., a date of admission to the hospital is then determined. In most community hospitals and for most types of surgical procedures, admission to the hospital is usually the afternoon of the day before the surgery is scheduled. Usually the admissions department is notified to expect the patient on day X for an operation on day Y. The admission department makes note of the admission date, and checks using their forecasting procedures to determine the probability of having a bed on day x.

2. Daily Procedures

Now let us see what happens on day X when the patients whose operations are on day Y are to be admitted.

TIME PERIOD	SITUATION
9:00 A.M.-1:00 P.M.	Discharges occur thus making beds available for new admissions. Some emergencies are admitted. Intra-hospital transfers (transfers between units) are also accomplished.
1:00 P.M.-3:00 P.M.	Scheduled patients arrive to be admitted. Some emergencies are admitted. Discharges occur. Patients are called in from waiting lists if beds are available.
3:00 P.M.-10:00 P.M.	The majority of emergencies are admitted. More discharges occur.
10:00 P.M.-9:00 A.M. The Next Day	Emergencies are admitted, if beds are available.

Some hospitals have a policy that all discharges are to be accomplished by 11:00 A.M. However, few hospitals have the necessary administrative controls to enforce the policy. Typically, 50% to 80% of the discharges occur by 11:00 A.M. in hospitals having such a policy.

3. Problems That Occur

Problems occur using this system in the following ways:

a. During the 1:00-3:00 P.M. period, scheduled patients are admitted provided that there are sufficient empty beds. Of course if there are insufficient beds, surgery cases will have difficulty being admitted. Please note the priority that the scheduled patients receive. They are admitted after the majority of discharges but before the majority of emergency patients arrive and before any non-scheduled elective patients are admitted.

b. During the 1:00-3:00 P.M. time period, if there are sufficient beds for the scheduled patients, consideration is given to non-scheduled elective patients that are on a waiting list. These patients are usually described in hospital policy manuals as patients needing to be admitted to the hospital within a certain number of days (usually 3-5 days). In most situations, hospital policy is not followed. Waiting list patients are not admitted within the stated number of days unless there are sufficient beds after scheduled patients are admitted and sufficient beds reserved for the arrival of emergency patients. "Sufficient" is the number of empty beds perceived by the admissions office to be necessary. The first obstacle in determining "sufficient" is that the majority of emergency patients arrive after the decision on the waiting list patients is made. Secondly, because the daily emergency arrivals vary widely from day to day, the admissions office may (and frequently does) make more allowance than is necessary for later emergency arrivals. This tendency reduces occupancy and delays the admission of the waiting list patients unnecessarily.

c. During the 3:00-10:00P.M. periods, emergencies arrive and are admitted if there have been sufficient discharges. If no bed is available, then the patient is kept in the emergency room until a bed becomes available, placed in a hall bed, or stabilized and sent to another hospital. Frequently when this situation occurs ambulances are requested to take patients to other hospitals. The patients that are kept in the emergency room or are put in hall beds are transferred as soon as possible.

4. Additional Problems

To complicate matters even more, the admissions officer has to contend with the following additional factors:

a. The number of scheduled patients often varies widely for different days of the week as well as for the same day of the week from week to week. This situation makes it very difficult for the admissions officer to plan his/her activities.

b. Discharges vary widely for different days of the week and for the same day of the week from week to week. Further, in hospitals that do surgery five days per week, patient discharges on the average are lower during the period Sunday through Wednesday whereas scheduled admissions are higher during this period. This increases the likelihood that scheduled patients will be cancelled, particularly on Wednesday and Thursday when the occupancy tends to peak. Thus, the number of beds that should be reserved for emergency admissions is different for every day of the week. Further, a decision to admit too many non-scheduled elective patients on, for example, Sunday, may result in elective surgical cancellations on the following Wednesday or Thursday thus making it very difficult for the admissions officer to learn by "cause and effect."

c. Emergencies vary widely -- again for different days of the week and for the same day from week to week. Since emergency admissions come from both the emergency room and also directly from doctors' offices, the difficulty of predicting the number of emergency admissions to expect is compounded. By occurring primarily during the day, direct emergency admissions only increase the probability that conflicts over available beds will occur with scheduled patients.
The net result of a, b, and c above is that there is so much uncertainty that it is very difficult to evolve the most appropriate and timely decisions. All of the above situations cause problems so that the admissions people may attempt to

influence the O.R. posting clerk to limit the number of scheduled surgeries. Also, the admissions office may try to admit waiting list patients after the dinner hour when the number of discharges is more precisely known. It gets more and more difficult, however to bring in waiting list patients as the day progresses. The late admission of these patients can cause problems for the ancillary service departments needed to perform first day of stay services for these patients. These admissions tend to help improve the occupancy situation because they reduce some of the uncertainty. However, they do not produce the maximum average occupanices and low numbers of cancellations and turnaways that are achievable using ASCS.

With the ASCS simulator, the management engineer and/or admissions officer can try out many different admission decision rules in a relatively short period of time. If the simulation of one set of decision rules is judged unacceptable, then the decision rules are changed and then resimulated. By simulating (replicating) 52 weeks of hospital operation, what is going to happen can be determined with a high degree of accuracy before it would ever happen. The change of decision rules and the simulation process occurs over and over again until an acceptable result is achieved.

C.   Teaching/Tertiary Hospital Admissions System

The teaching/tertiary hospital usually has one further complication - doctor allocations. Doctor allocation systems provide each service and/or clinical subspecialty with assigned beds and thus establishes a priority for those beds in times of conflict. The authors have examined two of these systems in detail and have concluded that the two non-ASCS systems are administrative methods appearing to solve a problem which in practice is very difficult to administer. The reasons are as follows:

1. Allocation System Based on Beds

If the allocation system is based on beds (for example, the neurosurgery service is assigned 20 beds), then the principal problem is to arrive at a reasonable method for admitting elective patients to these beds. The combination of length of stay, the number and variation of emergency admissions, together with the relatively small size of the bed allocation as well as excessive demand for beds by other services, makes the situation very difficult administratively. Either beds will remain empty due to attempts to avoid cancellations, or patients will frequently be placed in beds allocated to other services, thus defeating the objective of the allocation system.

2. Allocation System Based on Patient Days

This method involves allocating to each clinical service a number of patient days per month and the maintenance of cumulative totals for each service. At the end of each month the elective admission rates are adjusted according to which service is ahead or behind based on the cumulative totals. The reason that a unit may exceed its quota is the variation in the emergency rate and/or the need to keep the hospital full when another unit does not have enough patients to meet its quota. This system is more workable than the allocation of a specific number of beds; however, the "allocation" of patient days, which is not a physical entity like "beds," is sometimes hard to implement. Furthermore, it can create tensions among those physicians whose ability and need to admit elective patients change every month.

D.   The ASCS as an Allocation System

It is important to point out here that the ASCS system is in itself an allocation system. Each service or subservice can be allowed a given number of scheduled admissions over a period of time such as a week or a month. In addition, it has a provision to guarantee the admission of waiting list patients (hereafter called urgent) within a specific time frame as negotiated by administration and physicians. As a result, all urgents and emergency patients are admitted. Periodically, usually every six months, the historical patient arrival rates and average daily census (ADC) are compared with the forecasted rates and ADCs. The schedules are changed if major changes in patient mix are revealed. Thus, the ASCS has both a bed and patient day basis for its allocation. It emphasizes number of admissions on a daily basis and average numbers of beds used by a service on a periodic basis. The periodic review keeps the numbers used up to date and based on actual usage. Please note, that under the ASCS system, the allocation is accomplished by using the system. A separate system for allocations is not necessary. This greatly relieves the administrative problem.

E.   References

1.   Robinson, G.; Wing, P.; and Davis, L. "Computer Simulation of Hospital Patient Scheduling Systems," Health Services Research 3 (Summer 1968): 130-141.

2.   Subcommittee on Surgical Anesthesia, American Surgical Association, Report on the Operating Room Utilization Study, 1969.

CHAPTER III

A DESCRIPTION OF THE ASCS SYSTEM

A.   Introduction

At the admissions department level, the ASCS involves a series of numbers and rules that are to be used to make decisions at different times on each day. The system is designed basically as a "hand" system. This implies that for community hospitals, a computer is not necessary, although in some of the larger hospitals, the use of a computer is the recommended method of performing the computations involved.

B.   The Decision Numbers

The Decision Numbers are day of the week specific values, obtained via computer simulation of the hospital's admission process and patient flow dynamics. Once ascertained, these numbers are used by the hospital's admissions department on a daily basis to make objective decisions for the admissions process in a routine manner.

1. The Schedule Allowances

a. Elective Surgery

The admissions office and the operating room posting office are given a number for each day of the week representing the patients that they may advance schedule for admission for that day of the week.   These numbers, except under special circumstances to be discussed later, will not change from week to week. Typical of these numbers would be:

Sun	Mon	Tue	Wed	Thu	Fri	Sat
16	15	14	13	13	12	0

For some hospitals, further specification may also be made regarding the composition of each number in terms of each surgical specialty. For example, Sunday's 16 might imply 10 for general surgery, 2 for gynecology, 3 for orthopedics and 1 for neurosurgery.

Thus, on every Sunday, except during a holiday period, 16 surgical patients may be admitted for surgery on Monday or later. Generally, the O.R. posting clerk uses these numbers when talking to the physicians about scheduling dates for surgery. Without consultation with the admissions office, the posting clerk may go ahead and post surgery as long as these numbers are not exceeded. If he/she finds that there is good reason to exceed them, permission must be obtained from the admissions office. These numbers, when given to the O.R. posting clerk, are the numbers of beds that the admissions department guarantees will be available for the admission of elective surgery patients with a high probability (the degree of this probability is set by management policy). The probability is usually 97-99%.

Except at holiday periods, when it is desirable to change the numbers to account for no elective surgery on the holiday, the O.R. posting clerk can use the schedule for any day in the future. This property enables him/her to respond to a physician's request and to give alternate acceptable dates in the event that the O.R. clerk cannot fill the physician's first request.

Please note that the numbers are higher earlier in the week than toward the end of the week. This is typical of the pattern in most hospitals with or without the ASCS. It reflects the need to increase the census as quickly as possible after the weekend when few or no patients are admitted for surgery. This pattern, when there is high utilization of the O.R., means that the shorter O.R. procedures should be done earlier in the week and the longer procedures later in the week. With a typical O.R. utilization rate of approximately 50%, the differences in numbers between days of the week are not great enough to have much effect.

b. Elective Medicine

The same principle applies to elective medicals as well as elective surgicals except that the admissions department does all of the scheduling. Also, the number of elective medicals is usually much lower than that for elective surgery. The following is an example of an elective medical schedule:

Sun	Mon	Tue	Wed	Thu	Fri	Sat
2	2	2	1	2	3	4

Please note that the number of admissions increase toward the end of the week. This is to compensate, at least partially, for the fact that the majority of surgeries occur during the Monday to Friday period so that more beds are available toward the end of the week (don't forget, we usually want to keep occupancy as high as possible).

There are situations where no elective admissions are permitted (paid for by third parties) on weekends. If this is the case the schedule has to be changed accordingly. The ASCS simulator is very helpful here because, for the majority of cases, schedules can be established that do not result in an overall reduction in maximum average occupancy even though elective patients are not admitted on weekends.

2. The Census Reduction Allowance (CRA) and Cancellation Allowance (CA)

The CRA is a series of numbers (one for each day of the week) admissions personnel use in the determination of the number of urgent admissions to call in each day. The cancellation allowance (CA) is that minimum number of "empty beds" that must be saved for emergency admissions at the expense of cancelling scheduled admissions. If the empty beds are below the CA, then scheduled patients are cancelled until the number of empty beds equals the CA. Figure III-1 shows the relationship.

3. The Call-in Maximum Allowance (CMAX)

The CMAX is a day of the week specific ASCS allowance designed to place an upper limit on the number of patients that can be called in for admission. By restricting the maximum number of patients called in on a daily basis, the distribution of discharges is stabilized. For example, if the CRA is 36 as in Figure III-1 and CMAX is 5, then any time the number of empty beds is 41 or greater, only 5 patients may be called in.

C. The Decision Processes

Based upon the same simulation model used to obtain the decision numbers, sets of decision rules are constructed to define the hospital's admissions decision processes. Together the decision rules and decision numbers constitute the decision algorithm. It is this algorithm in conjunction with readily available data describing the hospital's present operating status that the admissions department uses daily to make the required decisions.

1. Decisions Concerning the "Empty Beds" Calculation

At a point in the day when the majority of discharges have occurred (usually 1 P.M. in a community hospital and 2-4 P.M. in a tertiary hospital) the number of usable empty beds are predicted using the following formula:

$$\#EMPTYBEDS = CAP - (CEN_{MID} + ADM_{EM} + ADM_{EL}) + DIS_1 + DIS_2$$

Where:

    a. CAP is the bed capacity of the hospital
    b. CEN_{MID} is the midnight census
    c. ADM_{EM} is the number of emergency admissions that have occurred since midnight
    d. ADM_{EL} is the number of elective patients scheduled for admission for the day
    e. DIS_1 is the number of discharges that occurred between midnight and the decision point

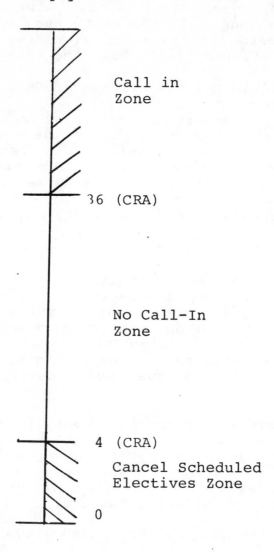

Figure III-1 An Example of the Relationship Between "Empty Beds", CRA and CA for a Particular Day of the Week

f. DIS_2 is the number of discharges expected to occur from the decision point until 9 A.M. the next day

In any given day at the final decision time, the admission officer can make three decisions concerning call-ins from the urgent category or the cancellation of previously scheduled patients. Using Figure III-1 as an example, these decisions are:

a. If the number of "empty beds" is greater than 36, then the admission officer should call in patients from the urgent list until there are 36 empty beds. For example, if there are 41 empty beds, then 5 patients should be called in (41-36=5). If the system uses a CMAX allowance, then the number to call in must be restricted to the value of the CMAX allowance for the day. Suppose that the CMAX were 3 in the example above. Then instead of calling in 5 patients, 3 patients would be called in. If the CMAX were 6, then 5 patients would still be called in.

b. If the number of "empty beds" were between 4 and 36, then the admissions officer would do nothing -- no call-ins.

c. If the number of empty beds were less than 4, then the admissions officer should cancel scheduled admissions (most likely surgery) until there were four empty beds. For example, if there were two empty beds, then 2 is the number of scheduled patients that should be rescheduled (4-2=2).

2. Typical Census Reduction Allowance (CRA)

The following is an example of a typical set of CRAs across the week.

Sun	Mon	Tue	Wed	Thu	Fri	Sat
40	32	27	23	21	38	65

The pattern of the numbers in this example is quite typical; i.e., high at the start of the week, rapidly decreasing to a low point on Thursday and then a sharp rise for Friday and Saturday. The strategy of this arrangement is as follows:

a. Sunday (40) -- There is usually an excess of empty beds going into the Sunday decision due to a normally low weekend census. It is true that this value (40) could be substantially lower and the hospital might not suffer on Sunday or Monday. However, for Tuesday through Thursday the probability of canceling and not having a bed for emergencies would be prohibitively high. At the same time, the probability of being able to call in any patients on Monday through Thursday would be very low. Therefore, the artifically high Sunday CRA serves to save beds for later in the week to reduce the likelihood of adverse situations and to promote the even distribution of call-ins across the week.

   b. Monday through Thursday -- As the week progresses, patients that have been given a fixed admission date have been admitted. As a result, fewer beds need to be saved. By Thursday, the CRA is at its lowest value for the week. It is no longer saving beds for patients scheduled on Friday and Saturday, but simply providing the needed safety margin for the evening's emergency admissions.

   c. Friday and Saturday -- At this point discharges are exceeding admission rates. As with Sunday, it would not jeopardize the situation for the weekend if the Friday and Saturday CRA values were significantly lower; however, if the CRA is set too low, surgical cancellations most likely would occur during the middle of the following week. Even with the high CRA values, call-ins can be made on Friday and Saturday because of the lack of scheduled surgery on Saturday and the increased discharges towards the end of the week.

There is a tendency for some administrators to view the size of the CRA with alarm because they conclude that the numbers represent the number of empty beds they will have. This view is not correct. The numbers represent the maximum numbers of beds that will be empty prior to admitting the evening's emergency admissions (assuming there are patients on the urgent waiting list). There will be many days when the "empty beds" will be in the no-call-in range (4-36 bed range in the Figure III-1 example).

   3. Typical Cancellation Allowance (CA)

The following is an example of typical CA's.

Sun	Mon	Tue	Wed	Thu	Fri	Sat
25	13	8	5	3	0	0

For a number of hospitals the ASCS does not utilize a CA; i.e., its values are zero for every day of the week. For those systems in which the CAs are used, the allowance can be quite high early in the week and then rapidly decrease, with the Friday and Saturday CA being zero. By design, over a period of time the distribution of cancellations across the week should not significantly differ from the distribution of patients scheduled across the week. Because a hospital will have a low weekend occupancy with respect to its overall occupancy, the high Sunday CA will not incur a greater number of cancellations on the average than any other day of the week.

The chances of having to cancel elective surgery are usually kept quite low. Thus, the probability that the number of "empty beds" would be below the CA point is low. The admissions officer should rarely find himself/herself having to use the CA.

4. Typical Call-In Maximum Allowances (CMAX)

To say that any one set of values is typical of the CMAX allowance would be misleading at best because the setting of this allowance is highly dependent on the hospital's objectives and limitations. The following is an example of CMAX allowances where weekend elective admissions are permitted and the objective is to provide for an even distribution of call-ins across the week.

SUN	MON	TUE	WED	THU	FRI	SAT
8	8	8	8	8	5	5

For units with large bed capacities the CMAX is usually set at the constant level for Sunday through Thursday and at approximately 60 percent of this weekday level for Friday and Saturday. The reasoning behind this strategy is that on the weekdays the system will utilize only 30 to 80 percent of the CMAX allowance (depending on the day of the week). On Friday and Saturday, however, it is not uncommon for 95 to 100 percent of the CMAX allowance to be consistently utilized.

In large teaching hospitals, a number of call-in streams can be utilized, each with its own set of CMAX allowances. For these situations the individual streams with their own CMAX serve to establish equity between the clinical services. This aspect as well as the use of the "Infinite CMAX" will be more fully discussed later in the chapter.

D. A Description of a Typical Community Hospital ASCS System

1. Introduction

The following pages contain the Decision Rules and Numbers that were used in a very successful implementation of the ASCS in a typical community hospital of 450 beds. The hospital, let us call it Community Hospital "ABC," can be viewed as typical because it has the clinical units that are most commonly found in community hospitals: Medical, Surgical, Obstetrics, and an ICU/CCU unit. The hospital's goals were to maximize occupancy with no more than 2 cancellations of scheduled admissions and 2 emergency turnaways on the average per month.

The hospital's ASCS was designed to make maximum use of the experience and capability of the admissions personnel. In order to accomplish this, there were three decision points:

1) 9 A.M. -- This first decision point was chosen so that the admissions officer could get an early look at the situation for the day and could make decisions on patient transfers so that they could be accomplished before the arrival of elective patients.

2) 11 A.M. -- This second decision point was designed to start the process of determining the existence of a high occupancy situation that could jeopardize the admission of scheduled and emergency patients. If the decision process indicated the existence of a sufficient number of empty beds, then patients could be called in. If the decision process indicated an insufficient number of beds to admit all patients scheduled for the day, then a "potential to cancel" situation was indicated and an adequate amount of time still existed to attempt to accelerate discharges in order to remedy the situation.

3) 1 P.M. -- This third and final decision point of the day was chosen because 80% of the day's discharges should have occurred by then and there was still time to call patients to come in during the afternoon or early evening.

2. The Decision Numbers

Figure III-2 contains the decision numbers given to the hospital's admissions department. These numbers were obtained using the ASCS Simulator.

	SU	MO	TU	WE	TH	FR	SA
MEDICAL SCHEDULED	0	0	0	1	1	1	0
SURGICAL SCHEDULED	12	11	11	9	7	5	0
GYN SCHEDULED	4	4	4	5	5	5	0
CRA	45	34	26	22	13	21	33
CA	4	4	3	3	2	2	0
CMAX	4	4	5	4	4	6	7

Figure III-2   The ASCS Decision Numbers for Community Hospital "ABC"

3. Admissions Decision Sheets

a. Preliminary Data -- Figure III-3 contains the preliminary data necessary to make the decisions for the day. This example is for a Wednesday. Because the decision numbers

Admissions Scheduling and Control System
Decision Sheets -- Hospital "ABC"

Date: 5/15/82   Day: Wednesday

	Sched. Allowances	# Scheduled		
MED:	[1]	1	CRA:	[22]
SURG:	[9]	9	CA:	[3]
GYN:	[5]	5		
			CMAX:	[4]
TOTALS:	[15]	15		

# of patients on urgent waiting list at 9 A.M. __6__

# of patients on Medical elective waiting list at 9 A.M. __2__

Figure III-3 Preliminary Data Sheet for Community Hospital "ABC"

III - 25

are the same for a given day each week, seven sets of decision sheets were prepared on which the constant decision numbers (appearing in braces) were printed on the forms. This saves time and minimizes the chances of errors. The constants are obtained from Figure III-2. The other numbers in Figure III-3 are part of the example and represent the day's entries by the admission department.

b. The 9 A.M. Decisions -- Figure III-4 illustrates the 9 A.M. Decision Work Sheet. Referring to Figure III-4, the following may be helpful.

Line 1. a. The number "2" represents the hospital's policy that two GYN patients can reside on OB.

Line 1. b. The unusable beds are those beds that cannot be used due to maintenance and/or contagious diseases.

Line 4. a. Forced transfers are the least severe patients in ICU/CCU that need to be transferred to MED/SURG to free up beds for arriving patients who need to be on the ICU/CCU unit immediately.

c. The 11 A.M. Decisions -- Figure III-5 illustrates the 11 A.M. Decision Work Sheets. Lines 1 through 4 are the same as the 9 A.M decisions except that the numbers have changed and the CA is used (line 3). Line 6 is a comment to remind the admissions officer to take extraordinary steps if subtotal B is negative. In this particular hospital the admissions officer did the following in order to prevent surgical cancellations:

1) Posted a red sign at the doctors' entrance indicating that empty beds were in short supply and that some surgeries would have to be cancelled if discharges did not increase.

2) Notified the Nursing Director's office so that he/she, in turn, could notify the head nurses. The head nurses, in turn were to monitor the bed situation and their floors and relay the bed need situation to the physicians wherever it was deemed appropriate.

3) Notified the emergency room. The intent here was to make sure that all emergency admissions were carefully screened.

Lines 7-12 are concerned with the 11 A.M. call-in decisions. In the example, Subtotal C is -14; thus no patients are to be called in. If patients are called in. we will exceed the allowable probability for cancellations and turnaways.

9 A.M. -- Decision on Transfers

1. Determine the # of available empty beds on MS at 9 A.M.

$$[2] + \frac{[328]}{\text{Med/Surg Capacity}} - \frac{300}{\text{9 a.m. MS census}} - \frac{2}{\text{9 a.m. GYN census on OB}} - \frac{6}{\text{9 a.m. # of MS unuseable beds}} = \frac{22}{}$$

2. Total # of scheduled patients

   Sched.Med. 1 + Sched.Surg 9 + Sched. Gyn 5 = (-)15

   Subtotal A = 7

3. If "Subtotal A" is positive, then patients may be transferred to MS. (The # of transfers may not exceed "Subtotal A")

From	Patients Needing to be Transferred	Patients Transferred
PEDS	2	2
EHA	0	0
ICU/CCU	4	4
OTHER		0
TOTALS	6	6

4. If "Subtotal A" is zero or negative, then defer transferring any patients into MS until after the 11 A.M. decision on transfers. (Note: Force transfers may occur at this time)

Figure III-4 -- The 9 A.M. Decision Work Sheet

11 A.M. -- Decision on Transfers

1. Determine the # of available empty beds on MS at 11 A.M.

$$[2] + \frac{[328]}{\substack{\text{Med/Surg} \\ \text{capacity}}} - \frac{296}{\substack{\text{11 A.M. MS} \\ \text{census}}} - \frac{2}{\substack{\text{11 A.M. GYN} \\ \text{census on OB}}} - \frac{6}{\substack{\text{11 A.M. \# of MS} \\ \text{unuseable beds}}} = \underline{26}$$

2. Total # of patients scheduled. . . . .   (-) 15

3. Cancellation allowance (CA). . . . .   (-) [3]

                                          Subtotal B =   8

4. If "Subtotal B" is positive, then patients may be transfered into MS (the number may not exceed "Subtotal B").

5. If "Subtotal B" is zero or negative, then defer transferring any patients into MS until after the 1 P.M. decision on transfers. Force transfers may be made at this time.

From	Patients Needing to be Transferred	Patients Transferred
PEDS	1	1
ICU/CCU	2	2
OTHER		
TOTALS	3	3

11 A.M. -- Potential Cancellations

6. If "Subtotal B" is negative, then its positive value represents the 11 A.M. potential number of scheduled patients to cancel. Initiate the procedure to accelerate MS discharges and determine the number of additional empty beds this will produce. Do not call in any patients at 11 A.M.

11 A.M. -- Decision on Call-Ins

7. Use "Subtotal B".   8

8. Use # of patients transferred to MS at 11 A.M. determination. . . . .   (-) 3

9. Cancellation allowance (CA). . . . .   (+) [3]

Figure III-5 The 11 A.M Decision Work Sheet

10. Census reduction allowance (CRA). . . . . (-)[22]

Subtotal C = - 14

11. If "Subtotal C" is positive, then call in patients such that the number called in does not exceed "Subtotal C" or the CMAX Allowance. (Call in patients on urgent waiting list first.)

List	11 A.M Waiting List Length	# of Patients Called in at 11 A.M.
Urgent	6	0
Elec. Med.	2	0
Totals	8	0

12. If "Subtotal C" is zero or negative, then do not call in any patients until after 1 P.M. decision on call-ins.

Figure III-5   The 11 A.M. Decision Work Sheet (Continued)

<u>1 P.M. -- Decision on Transfers</u>

1. Determine the # of available empty beds on MS at 1 P.M.

$$[2] + \frac{[328]}{\substack{\text{Med/Surg} \\ \text{capacity}}} - \frac{294}{\substack{\text{1 pm MS} \\ \text{census}}} - \frac{2}{\substack{\text{1 pm GYN} \\ \text{census on OB}}} - \frac{6}{\substack{\text{1 pm # of MS} \\ \text{unuseable beds}}} = \frac{28}{}$$

2. Total # of scheduled patients not yet admitted. . . =(-) 15

3. Total # of patients called-in at 11 A.M., but not
   yet admitted. (-) 0

4. Cancellation allowance. . . . . (-) [3]

                                        Subtotal D = 10

From	Patients Needing to be Transferred	Patients Transferred
PEDS	0	0
ICU/CCU	0	0
OTHER	0	0
TOTALS	0	0

<u>1 P.M. -- Decision on Cancellations</u>

5. If "Subtotal D" is negative, then its positive value represents
   the 1 P.M. potential number of patients to cancel. Determine if
   any additional discharges will occur and then proceed with lines
   6 through 8.

6. 1 P.M. number of patients to cancel
   (Enter the positive value of Subtotal D)
                                        (+) 3

7. Empty beds expected by latest inquiry
   for expected late
                                        (-) 2

                     Subtotal E =   1

8. If "subtotal E" is greater than zero, then subtotal E represents
   the number of scheduled patients to cancel. Do not call in any
   patients.

<u>1 P.M. -- Decision on Call-Ins</u>

9. Use "Subtotal D"   (+) 10

10. Cancellation allowance (CA)   (+) [3]

Figure III-6 The 1 P.M. Decision Work Sheet

III - 30

11. Use number of patients transferred to MS at
    1 P.M. determination   (-)   0

12. Census Reduction Allowance (CRA)   ·   (-) [22]

                                 Subtotal F =   - 9

13. Determine the # of additional patients which could have been
    scheduled:

Type	Schedule Allowance	Patients Scheduled	# of Additional Patients Which Could Have Been Scheduled
MED	1	1	0
SURG	9	9	0
GYN	5	5	0
TOTALS	15 -	15 =	0

14. Use Med. Max. Call-In Allowance . (+)   [3]

15. Use the total number of patients
    called in at 11 A.M. . . . . . . (-)   0

16. The 1 P.M. CMAX. . . . . =   3
    (The sum of the number of additional
    patients which could have been
    scheduled plus the days Call-in
    Maximum allowance minus the number
    of patients called in at 11 A.M.)

17. If both "Subtotal F" and "The 1 P.M. CMAX" are positive, then
    call in patients such that the 1 P.M. number of call-ins does
    not exceed either "Subtotal F" or "The 1 P.M. CMAX" (Call in
    patients on the urgent waiting list first.)

List	1 P.M. Waiting List Length	# of Patients Called in at 1 P.M.
Urgent	6	0
Elec. Med.	2	0
Totals	8	0

Figure III-6   The 1 P.M. Decision Work Sheet (Continued)

d. The 1 P.M. Decisions -- Figure III-6 illustrates the 1 P.M. Decision Work Sheets. As mentioned previously, 1 P.M. was chosen as the final decision time for the day because a large number of the discharges would have had occurred due to an effective 11 A.M. discharge time and there would still time to call in patients if it is deemed necessary. Also, by telling scheduled elective patients to come in between 2 P.M. and 3 P.M., there would be sufficient time to notify patients before they leave home if it became necessary to cancel.

Lines 1-4 of Figure III-6 are concerned with the 1 P.M. decisions on transfers. Usually by this time, all transfers have been accomplished unless occupancy is very high. If the need for additional transfers arises between 11 A.M. and 1 P.M., either because of late discharges or because of increased emphasis on discharges caused by the extraordinary procedures of the admissions officer due to the 11 A.M. decision work sheet calculations, it may be possible to transfer the patients at this time. In this example, there is room to transfer patients, but all transfers have occurred.

Lines 5-8, Figure III-6 are the decision steps that determine if it will be necessary to cancel surgery. Since subtotal D in our example is positive (10), no surgical cancellations are necessary. Suppose, however, that subtotal D were -3, then 3 would be entered on line 6 as illustrated. Line 7 is an indication to the admissions officer that he/she should query the floors to make sure that there are no late discharges that have not had time to clear the discharge procedures. Also, a patient could be leaving, but be held in a bed until someone could come to pick him/her up. Suppose two such patients were located. Subtotal E would then be 1 which is the number of scheduled admissions that would have to be canceled and rescheduled on another day. Please keep in mind that cancellations rarely happen using the system. The average number for this hospital was 2 per month.

Lines 9 through 12 are the decision rules for determining the number of call-ins. If we use our original value of subtotal D (10), then subtotal F is -9 as illustrated. Lines 13 to 16 are to determine if the CMAX (4) can be increased if all of the schedule slots were not used. All the schedule slots were used as illustrated, and therefore the 1 P.M. CMAX (line 16) is not increased over its original value.

Line 17 contains the instructions concerning the number of patients to call-in. In our example the value of line 17, the 1 P.M. call in maximum is 3; but subtotal F is -9, so no patients should be called in. Suppose subtotal F were +2. Then according to line 17 we would call in 2 patients. If subtotal F were 6, we would call in only 3 patients because we would be constrained by the 1 P.M. CMAX.

Comments of the Admissions Officers Concerning the Forms

Admissions officers frequently say that the system looks complicated and that the meaning of the words CRA, CA and CMAX are difficult to understand. However, the fears quickly disappear after the forms are used for a few days. The usual procedure is for the admissions officers to attempt to fill in the forms, but to have available a management engineer or other support person to check calculations and answer any questions.

After two or three days, the admissions officers begin to memorize the forms and to fill in only those portions that are dictated by the daily situation. For example, if the occupancy is low on a weekend, the cancellation calculations are skipped.

4. Problems That the Admissions Personnel Have Experienced

During the first week of operation two problems appear that should be mentioned. The first is that the admissions clerical staff that work weekends have to be properly trained so that errors do not occur when ASCS advisors may not be available. The second is that the requirement to use negative numbers occasionally causes difficulty. One admission group has had to conduct a special class on negative numbers in order to solve the problem.

E. The Admission Decision Forms for a Teaching Hospital

1. Introduction

Although the original ASCS system was specifically designed to be used in community hospitals, more interest has been shown by large teaching hospitals. The primary differences between the large teaching hospitals and community hospitals with respect to patient flows are that in the teaching hospitals:

    a. There are a large number of clinical units devoted to the delivery of care associated with the clinical specialty.

    b. There are many more transfers between units during patients' hospital stay.

    c. Beds are allocated for each of the clinical services and there may exist rules regulating the use of certain beds for emergency admissions and/or off-service patients.

    d. There are more restrictions concerning the use of Intensive Care units for acute patients.

    e. The number of scheduled elective streams are greater because surgery is usually performed by a number of surgical specialties.

Experience has indicated that all of the above factors can be handled by the ASCS Simulator; however, the resulting decision rules become more lengthy and to some extent more complex.

2. Teaching Hospital Description

For purposes of an example, a 781-bed teaching hospital has been chosen. This hospital, let us call it Teaching Hospital "XYZ,"*has 7 clinical units, a 20-bed swing unit with no clinical designation, and a number of intensive care units that are not permitted to handle any patient overflow from acute units.

3. Typical Decision Numbers

Figure III-7 contains the decision numbers that the admissions officer is to use with the system. Please note that there are many more scheduled allowances, a larger number of CMAX allowances, and an Adjustment Factor for MedB #2 Call-Ins which were not a part of the community hospital example.

4. Admission Decision Sheets

a. The 9 A.M. Decision Tables

Figure III-8 illustrates the 9 A.M. decision rules, which are called Decision Tables because of their tabular appearance. For lines 1 to 17, the admissions officer is asked to fill in the appropriate numbers and to do the necessary calculations. Each cell not containing X's is to be filled in. Every attempt has been made to make the instructions as self-explanatory as possible, thus eliminating the need to refer to a separate instruction manual which could divert the user's attention and introduce errors. Transfer decisions, which were emphasized in the community hospital decisions, are incorporated in lines 9 and 13. The policy of this hospital regarding transfers is that they will have first priority and the decision tables reflect this policy. However, by taking into consideration the minimum number of discharges expected for the day on line 10, some call-ins may be possible in low-occupancy situations early in the day. These numbers appear in Table #1.A. of Figure III-9. The use of the 9 A.M. decision tables accomplishes two important purposes:

1. 9 A.M. represents the start of the hospital's admission day (in terms of the ASCS). As such, it initiates the day's ASCS data collection.

2. After a few weeks of using all of the system's decision tables, the admissions officer will realize that the value on Line 17 will generally be below the CRA and occasionally negative (implying no 9 A.M. call-ins). However, the magnitude of this number soon becomes a valuable indicator that can be used to gauge the difficulty to be expected for the rest of the day.

Please note that the first page of the 9 A.M. decision tables is designed to be filled in from left to right, i.e., each line is filled in starting with column 1 and going across the

---

*XYZ hospital is Harper Hospital, Detroit, MI. Reproduced with permission.

HOSPITAL "XYZ"

TABLE #1 -- ASCS TABLE OF ALLOWANCES

SERVICE	ALLOWANCE	SUN	MON	TUE	WED	THU	FRI	SAT	TOTAL
MED_A	SCHED	2	2	2	3	1	0	0	10
MED_B	SCHED	5	2	2	2	2	2	0	15
GEN_SUR	SCHED	17	13	12	12	9	4	0	67
ENT	SCHED	5	5	4	3	4	0	0	21
GYN	SCHED	1	0	1	1	1	0	0	4
OPT	SCHED	6	5	3	6	4	0	0	24
ORT	SCHED	4	4	4	3	3	0	0	18
URO	SCHED	5	5	3	3	2	0	0	18
ONC_A	SCHED	1	1	1	1	1	1	0	6
ONC_B	SCHED	1	0	0	0	0	0	0	1
NEU	SCHED	2	1	0	0	1	1	1	6
NSU	SCHED	3	2	2	2	1	0	0	10
FPR	SCHED	0	0	1	0	0	0	0	1
CANCELLATION ALLOWANCE	CAN	37	14	12	11	10	0	0	
CENSUS REDUCTION ALLOWANCE	CRA	40	30	25	20	14	46	78	
MED_B	CMAX_#1	2	2	2	2	3	4	5	
SURG (TOTAL)	CMAX	3	4	3	2	2	2	2	
MED_A	CMAX	4	4	4	3	3	3	3	
ONC_A	CMAX	4	4	5	5	4	4	4	
NEU_NSU	CMAX	4	3	3	3	2	1	1	
ONC_B	CMAX	1	1	1	1	1	1	1	
FPR	CMAX	2	1	1	1	1	1	1	
MEDB	CMAX_#2	99	99	99	99	99	99	99	
ADJUSTMENT FACTOR FOR MEDB_#2 CALLINS		3	0	2	6	6	6	6	

Figure III-7 ASCS Decision Numbers for Teaching Hospital "XYZ"

TODAY'S DATE: _____   DAY OF THE WEEK: _____

PREPARED BY: _____

		COL 1	COL 2	COL 3	COL 4	COL 5	COL 6	COL 7	COL 8	COL 9
LINE#	ITEM	MED_B	SURG	MED_A	ONC_A	NEU_NSU	ONC_B	FPR	SWING	ACUTE TOTALS
1	TODAY'S EMPTY SCHEDULE SLOTS								XXXX	XXXX
2	TODAY'S CALLIN MAXIMUMS (CMAX) (FROM THE TABLE OF ASCS ALLOWANCES -- TABLE #1)								XXXX	XXXX
3	THE 9AM CALLIN MAXIMUMS (LINE 1 + LINE 2)								XXXX	XXXX
4	UNIT CAPACITY	91	304	166	79	88	30	14	21	XXXX
5	BEDS OUT OF SERVICE ON UNIT									XXXX
6	SERVICEABLE BEDS ON UNIT (LINE 4 - LINE 5)									XXXX
7	9AM CENSUS ON UNIT									XXXX
8	# OF SERVICEABLE EMPTY BEDS ON UNIT AT 9AM (LINE 6 - LINE 7)	(+)	(+)	(+)	(+)	(+)	(+)	(+)	(+)	(=)
9	ENTER THE EXPECTED # OF TRANSFER REQUESTS FROM ACUTE TO ICU BETWEEN 9AM TODAY AND 9AM TOMORROW	XXXX	XXXX	XXXX	XXXX	XXXX	XXXX	XXXX	XXXX	
10	ENTER THE MINIMUM EXPECTED NUMBER OF PATIENTS TO BE DISCHARGED BETWEEN 9AM TODAY AND 9AM TOMORROW (FROM TABLE #1.A.)	XXXX	XXXX	XXXX	XXXX	XXXX	XXXX	XXXX	XXXX	
11	SUBTOTAL (LINE 8 + LINE 9 + LINE 10)	XXXX	XXXX	XXXX	XXXX	XXXX	XXXX	XXXX	XXXX	
12	ENTER THE # OF PATIENTS SCHEDULED FOR ADMISSION TODAY	(+)	(+)	(+)	(+)	(+)	(+)	(+)	XXXX	(=)
13	ENTER THE EXPECTED # OF TRANSFER REQUESTS FROM ICU TO ACUTE BETWEEN 9AM TODAY AND 9AM TOMORROW	XXXX	XXXX	XXXX	XXXX	XXXX	XXXX	XXXX	XXXX	
14	SUBTOTAL (LINE 12 + LINE 13)	XXXX	XXXX	XXXX	XXXX	XXXX	XXXX	XXXX	XXXX	
15	EMPTY BED COUNT DIFFERENCE (LINE 11 - LINE 14)	XXXX	XXXX	XXXX	XXXX	XXXX	XXXX	XXXX	XXXX	
16	CENSUS REDUCTION ALLOWANCE (CRA) (FROM THE TABLE OF ASCS ALLOWANCES -- TABLE #1)	XXXX	XXXX	XXXX	XXXX	XXXX	XXXX	XXXX	XXXX	
17	# OF ASCS EMPTY BEDS AVAILABLE FOR 9AM CALLINS (LINE 15 - LINE 16)	XXXX	XXXX	XXXX	XXXX	XXXX	XXXX	XXXX	XXXX	

NOTE #1: "ACUTE TOTALS" IS USED IN THE DECISION TABLES TO DENOTE EITHER BEDS OR PATIENTS ASSOCIATED WITH THE SERVICES MED_A, MED_B, SURG, ONC_A, ONC_B, NEU_NSU, FPR AND THE SWING UNIT.

NOTE #2: WHEN "(+)" APPEARS IN THE BOX FORMED BY A COLUMN AND ROW, THEN ITS VALUE IS TO BE INCLUDED IN THE SUMMATION TO BE PLACED IN COLUMN #9 OF THE ROW. BOXES NOT CONTAINING "(+)" MUST BE OMITTED FROM THE ROW'S SUMMATION.

Figure III-8   The 9 A.M. Decision Tables

                                              9AM DECISION TABLE

TODAY'S DATE: _____   DAY OF THE WEEK: _____

PREPARED BY:
            _____

PROCEDURE FOR CALCULATING # OF PATIENTS TO CALLIN:
1. PROCESS THE COLUMN FOR MEDB_#1 LINE 18 THRU LINE 22.
2. PROCESS THE COLUMN FOR SURG LINE 18 THRU LINE 22.
3. PROCESS THE COLUMN FOR MED_A LINE 18 THRU LINE 22.
4. PROCESS THE COLUMN FOR ONC_A LINE 18 THRU LINE 22.
5. PROCESS THE COLUMN FOR NEU_NSU LINE 18 THRU LINE 22.
6. PROCESS THE COLUMN FOR ONC_B LINE 18 THRU LINE 22.
6. PROCESS THE COLUMN FOR FPR LINE 18 THRU LINE 24.
8. PROCESS THE COLUMN FOR MEDB_#2 LINE 18 THRU LINE 22.

LINE#	ITEM	COL 1 MEDB_#1	COL 2 SURG	COL 3 MED_A	COL 4 ONC_A	COL 5 NEU_NSU	COL 6 ONC_B	COL 7 FPR	COL 8 MEDB_#2
18	# OF ASCS EMPTY BEDS REMAINING FOR CALLINS (ENTER IN COL #1 THE VALUE FROM LINE 17, COL #9)								
19	ENTER THE SERVICE'S CALLIN WAITING LIST LENGTH AT 9AM (NOTE FOR MEDB_#2: TAKE INTO ACCOUNT THE # OF PATIENTS TO BE CALLED IN FOR MEDB_#1)								
20	ENTER THE 9AM CALLIN MAXIMUM FOR THE SERVICE (FROM LINE 3)								??
21	# OF PATIENTS TO CALLIN AT 9AM (TAKE THE MINIMUM OF LINE 18, LINE 19 AND LINE 20) IF THE RESULT IS NEGATIVE, THEN ENTER '0')								
22	# OF EMPTY BEDS REMAINING AFTER CALLINS (LINE 18 - LINE 21) (EXCEPT FOR FPR AND MEDB_#2: COPY THE VALUE CALCULATED TO LINE 18 IN THE NEXT COLUMN)								

IF THE COLUMN LAST PROCESSED ON LINE 22 WAS NOT FOR "FPR" OR "MEDB_#2", THEN CONTINUE WITH THE NEXT COLUMN ON LINE 18.

LINE#	ITEM							FPR	MEDB_#2
23	ENTER TODAY'S ADJUSTMENT FACTOR FOR MEDB_#2 CALLINS (FROM THE TABLE OF ASCS ALLOWANCES -- TABLE #1)	/////////	/////////	/////////	/////////	/////////	/////////		/////////
24	ADJUST # OF EMPTY BEDS REMAINING FOR MEDB_#2 CALLINS (LINE 22 - LINE 23: PLACE THE VALUE HERE AND IN COLUMN #8 OF LINE 18).	/////////	/////////	/////////	/////////	/////////	/////////		/////////

NOTE: THE PROCEDURE TO FOLLOW WHEN PHONING PATIENTS TO BE CALLED IN:
ALWAYS CALL IN THE PATIENTS WHO HAVE BEEN WAITING THE LONGEST FOR ADMISSION UNLESS OTHERWISE INSTRUCTED. DO THIS UNTIL ONE OF THE FOLLOWING TWO CONDITIONS OCCUR:
1. ALL PATIENTS ON THE SERVICE'S WAITING LIST HAVE BEEN PHONED.
2. THE NUMBER OF CONFIRMATIONS BY PHONE IS THE SAME AS THE # OF PATIENTS TO CALL IN (ON LINE 21).

Figure III-8   The 9 A.M. Decision Tables (Continued)

HOSPITAL "XYZ"

TABLE #1.A.:   MINIMUM EXPECTED NUMBER OF PATIENTS
TO BE .DISCHARGED BETWEEN 9 AM TODAY AND 9 AM TOMORROW

SUN	MON	TUE	WED	THU	FRI	SAT
24	36	50	56	47	71	59

Figure III-9 Tables of·Minimum Expected Discharges for 9 A.M.
ASCS Decision Tables (line 10) for Teaching Hospital "XYZ"

line to column 9. Column 9 is the totals column which is the only row cell used after line 11. In practice the decision tables are printed for each day of the week with the appropriate values from Figure III-7 printed on them. This reduces the chances of clerical error and reduces the time necessary to complete the calculations.

b. The 1 P.M. Decision Tables

The 1 P.M. decision tables (Figure III-10) are essentially an updating of the 9 A.M. decision tables. The choice of 1 P.M. as the second decision point is primarily due to the fact that the hospital experiences late discharges. By 1 P.M. a sufficient number of discharges has occurred to enable estimation of the total number of discharges that can be expected for the day. In turn, there is still sufficient time before the final decision point to take any required extraordinary action.

Lines 1-3 are used to determine the 1 P.M. call-in maximums which are a modification of the 9 A.M. CMAX due to any patients called in at 9 A.M. Lines 4-10 are essentially the same for all three of the decision tables. Lines 11-21 are to determine if there is a potential for scheduled cancellations. Line 18 is of particular interest because it involves the use of a look-up table (Figure III-11). Table 2 contains a day of the week specific estimate of the minimum discharges that are likely to occur based on the discharges that have already occurred between 9 A.M. and 1 P.M. These values were obtained by analyzing the time of discharge of patients for each day of the week for a period of several months. If line 21 indicates patient cancellations, then this is a warning that one or more cancellations are possible. Since the discharges after 1 P.M. are conservatively predicted, the probability of a cancellation is not high but is a possibility. In other words, if no cancellations are predicted, then there is a very high probability that none will occur. If a cancellation is predicted, it may not occur, but the admissions officer is forewarned of potential trouble. He/she may elect to take the extraordinary procedures as instructed on Line 22 which have also been described earlier in this chapter. Line 22 also contains the instruction that if cancellations are predicted from line 21, that the next section should not be used because no call-ins will be made.

Lines 23 to 33 are for the call-in decisions. The format of the table changes beginning with line 27. For lines 27 to 33 the numbers are filled in by going down column 1 and repeating this procedure for each column until column 7, where lines 32 and 33 are filled in, before returning to line 27 of column 8. The call-in calculations for a teaching hospital are usually more complex because if call-ins can be made, we want to call patients in for each of the clinical services rather than call all of the patients in for the same service. This serves to allocate the patients between services. After the allocation has been accomplished, there is an overall call-in stream (any unit, Col. 8) that can be used for patients from any service. The any unit call-in stream is important because it enables the census to be

TODAY'S DATE: _____   DAY OF THE WEEK: _____

PREPARED BY: _____

LINE#	ITEM	COL 1 MED_B	COL 2 SURG	COL 3 MED_A	COL 4 ONC_A	COL 5 NEU_NSU	COL 6 ONC_B	COL 7 FPR	COL 8 SWING	COL 9 ACUTE TOTALS
1	THE 9AM CALLIN MAXIMUMS (FROM PAGE #1, LINE #3)								XXXXXX	XXXXXX
2	ENTER THE # OF PATIENTS SUCCESSFULLY CALLED IN BETWEEN 9AM AND 1PM								XXXXXX	XXXXXX
3	THE 1PM CALLIN MAXIMUMS (LINE 1 - LINE 2)								XXXXXX	XXXXXX
4	UNIT CAPACITY	91	304	156	79	88	30	13	20	XXXXXX
5	BEDS OUT OF SERVICE ON UNIT									XXXXXX
6	SERVICEABLE BEDS ON UNIT (LINE 4 - LINE 5)									XXXXXX
7	1PM CENSUS ON UNIT									XXXXXX
8	# OF SERVICEABLE EMPTY BEDS ON UNIT AT 1PM (LINE 6 - LINE 7)	(+)	(+)	(+)	(+)	(+)	(+)	(+)	(+)	(=)
9	ENTER THE EXPECTED # OF TRANSFER REQUESTS FROM ACUTE TO ICU BETWEEN 1PM TODAY AND 9AM TOMORROW	XXXXXX	XXXXXX	XXXXXX	XXXXXX	XXXXXX	XXXXXX	XXXXXX	XXXXXX	
10	SUBTOTAL (LINE 8 + LINE 9)	XXXXXX	XXXXXX	XXXXXX	XXXXXX	XXXXXX	XXXXXX	XXXXXX	XXXXXX	
11	ENTER THE # OF PATIENTS SCHEDULED FOR ADMISSION TODAY BUT NOT YET ADMITTED	(+)	(+)	(+)	(+)	(+)	(+)	(+)	XXXXXX	(=)
12	ENTER THE # OF PATIENTS SUCCESSFULLY CALLED IN TODAY BUT NOT YET ADMITTED	(+)	(+)	(+)	(+)	(+)	(+)	(+)	XXXXXX	(=)
13	ENTER THE EXPECTED # OF TRANSFER REQUESTS FROM ICU TO ACUTE BETWEEN 1PM TODAY AND 9AM TOMORROW	XXXXXX	XXXXXX	XXXXXX	XXXXXX	XXXXXX	XXXXXX	XXXXXX	XXXXXX	
14	SUBTOTAL (LINE 11 + LINE 12 + LINE 13)	XXXXXX	XXXXXX	XXXXXX	XXXXXX	XXXXXX	XXXXXX	XXXXXX	XXXXXX	
15	EMPTY BED COUNT DIFFERENCE (LINE 10 - LINE 14)	XXXXXX	XXXXXX	XXXXXX	XXXXXX	XXXXXX	XXXXXX	XXXXXX	XXXXXX	

NOTE #1: "ACUTE TOTALS" IS USED IN THE DECISION TABLES TO DENOTE EITHER BEDS OR PATIENTS ASSOCIATED WITH THE SERVICES MED_A, MED_B, SURG, ONC_A, ONC_B, NEU_NSU, FPR AND THE SWING UNIT.

NOTE #2: WHEN "(+)" APPEARS IN THE BOX FORMED BY A COLUMN AND ROW, THEN ITS VALUE IS TO BE INCLUDED IN THE SUMMATION TO BE PLACED IN COLUMN #9 OF THE ROW. BOXES NOT CONTAINING "(+)" MUST BE OMITTED FROM THE ROW'S SUMMATION.

Figure III-10 The 1 P.M. Decision Tables

TODAY'S DATE: _____   DAY OF THE WEEK: _____

PREPARED BY: _____

LINE#	ITEM	COL 1 MED_B	COL 2 SURG	COL 3 MED_A	COL 4 ONC_A	COL 5 NEU_NSU	COL 6 ONC_B	COL 7 FPR	COL 8 SWING	COL 9 ACUTE TOTALS
16	REENTER THE VALUE FROM LINE 15	XXXXXXXX	XXXXXXXX	XXXXXXXX	XXXXXXXX	XXXXXXXX	XXXXXXXX	XXXXXXXX	XXXXXXXX	
17	ENTER THE # OF PATIENTS DISCHARGED OR EXPIRED TODAY BETWEEN 9AM AND 1PM	(+)	(+)	(+)	(+)	(+)	(+)	(+)	(+)	(=)
18	FOR POTENTIAL CANCELLATION DECISION: ENTER THE EXPECTED # OF EMPTY BEDS TO BECOME AVAILABLE BETWEEN 1PM TODAY AND 9AM TOMORROW DUE TO DISCHARGES (BASED ON LINE 17 AND TABLE #2)									
19	EXPECTED # OF SERVICEABLE EMPTY BEDS FOR POTENTIAL CANCELLATION DECISION (LINE 16 + LINE 18)									
20	ENTER THE CANCELLATION ALLOWANCE (CAN) (FROM THE TABLE OF ASCS ALLOWANCES -- TABLE #1)									
21	THE EXPECTED # OF ASCS EMPTY BEDS FOR THE POTENTIAL CANCELLATION DECISION (LINE 19 - LINE 20)									

| 22 | IF THE VALUE OF LINE 21 IS NEGATIVE, THEN IT REPRESENTS THE NUMBER OF POTENTIAL CANCELLATIONS FOR THOSE PATIENTS NOT YET ADMITTED WHO WERE SCHEDULED OR CALLED IN FOR ADMISSION TODAY. IF THIS IS THE CASE, THEN:
 A. WARN THE ADMISSIONS OFFICE SUPERVISOR OF THE SITUATION SO THAT ACCELERATED DISCHARGE PROCEDURES AND SPECIAL TRANSFER PROCEDURES CAN BE INVOKED TO INSURE THAT THE NECESSARY EMPTY BEDS WILL BE AVAILABLE TO AVOID CANCELLATIONS.
     1. ACCELERATED DISCHARGE PROCEDURES CONSIST OF ALERTING THE SERVICES AND PHYSICIANS OF THE SITUATION AND REQUESTING THAT PATIENTS THAN CAN BE SAFELY DISCHARGED TODAY BE DISCHARGED AS SOON AS POSSIBLE. REQUEST FROM NURSING ADMINISTRATION THAT A LIST OF ALL DISCHARGES KNOWN TO BE OCCURING AFTER 2PM BE MADE AVAILABLE.
     2. SPECIAL TRANSFER PROCEDURES CONSIST OF DELAYING THE TRANSFER OF PATIENTS FROM ICU BEDS TO ACUTE BEDS AT THIS TIME.
 B. DISCONTINUE PROCESSING THE 1PM DECISION TABLES. DO NOT CALL IN ANY PATIENTS AT THIS TIME. | | | | | | | | | |

23	FOR CALLIN DECISION: ENTER THE EXPECTED # OF EMPTY BEDS TO BECOME AVAILABLE BETWEEN 1PM TODAY AND 9AM TOMORROW DUE TO DISCHARGES (BASED ON LINE 17 AND TABLE #3)									
24	EXPECTED # OF SERVICEABLE EMPTY BEDS FOR CALLIN DECISION (LINE 16 + LINE 23)									
25	CENSUS REDUCTION ALLOWANCE (CRA) (FROM THE TABLE OF ASCS ALLOWANCES -- TABLE #1)									
26	# OF ASCS EMPTY BEDS AVAILABLE FOR 1PM CALLINS (LINE 24 - LINE 25)									

NOTE #1: "ACUTE TOTALS" IS USED IN THE DECISION TABLES TO DENOTE EITHER BEDS OR PATIENTS ASSOCIATED WITH THE SERVICES MED_A, MED_B, SURG, ONC_A, ONC_B, NEU_NSU, FPR AND THE SWING UNIT.
NOTE #2: WHEN "(+)" APPEARS IN THE BOX FORMED BY A COLUMN AND ROW, THEN ITS VALUE IS TO BE INCLUDED IN THE SUMMATION TO BE PLACED IN COLUMN #9 OF THE ROW. BOXES NOT CONTAINING "(+)" MUST BE OMITTED FROM THE ROW'S SUMMATION.

Figure III-10   The 1 P.M. Decision Tables (Continued)

1PM DECISION TABLE

TODAY'S DATE: _____   DAY OF THE WEEK: _____

PREPARED BY:
      _____

PROCEDURE FOR CALCULATING # OF PATIENTS TO CALLIN:
1. PROCESS THE COLUMN FOR MEDB_#1 LINE 27 THRU LINE 31.
2. PROCESS THE COLUMN FOR SURG LINE 27 THRU LINE 31.
3. PROCESS THE COLUMN FOR MED_A LINE 27 THRU LINE 31.
4. PROCESS THE COLUMN FOR ONC_A LINE 27 THRU LINE 31.
5. PROCESS THE COLUMN FOR NEU_NSU LINE 27 THRU LINE 31.
6. PROCESS THE COLUMN FOR ONC_B LINE 27 THRU LINE 31.
6. PROCESS THE COLUMN FOR FPR LINE 27 THRU LINE 33.
8. PROCESS THE COLUMN FOR MEDB_#2 LINE 27 THRU LINE 31.

LINE#	ITEM	COL 1 MEDB_#1	COL 2 SURG	COL 3 MED_A	COL 4 ONC_A	COL 5 NEU_NSU	COL 6 ONC_B	COL 7 FPR	COL 8 MEDB_#2
27	# OF ASCS EMPTY BEDS REMAINING FOR CALLINS (ENTER IN COL #1 THE VALUE FROM LINE 26, COL #9)								
28	ENTER THE SERVICE'S CALLIN WAITING LIST LENGTH AT 1PM (NOTE FOR MEDB_#2: TAKE INTO ACCOUNT THE # OF PATIENTS TO BE CALLED IN FOR MEDB_#1)								
29	ENTER THE 1PM CALLIN MAXIMUM FOR THE SERVICE (FROM LINE 3)								99
30	# OF PATIENTS TO CALLIN AT 1PM (TAKE THE MINIMUM OF LINE 27, LINE 28 AND LINE 29: IF THE RESULT IS NEGATIVE, THEN ENTER '0')								
31	# OF EMPTY BEDS REMAINING AFTER CALLINS (LINE 27 - LINE 30) (EXCEPT FOR FPR AND MEDB_#2, COPY THE VALUE CALCULATED TO LINE 27 IN THE NEXT COLUMN)								

IF THE COLUMN LAST PROCESSED ON LINE 31 WAS NOT FOR 'FPR' OR 'MEDB_#2', THEN CONTINUE WITH THE NEXT COLUMN ON LINE 27.

LINE#	ITEM	COL 1	COL 2	COL 3	COL 4	COL 5	COL 6	COL 7	COL 8
32	ENTER TODAY'S ADJUSTMENT FACTOR FOR MEDB_#2 CALLINS (FROM THE TABLE OF ASCS ALLOWANCES -- TABLE #1)	//////	//////	//////	//////	//////	//////		//////
33	ADJUST # OF EMPTY BEDS REMAINING FOR MEDB_#2 CALLINS (LINE 31 - LINE 32: PLACE THE VALUE HERE AND IN COLUMN #8 OF LINE 27).	//////	//////	//////	//////	//////	//////		//////

NOTE: THE PROCEDURE TO FOLLOW WHEN PHONING PATIENTS TO BE CALLED IN:
ALWAYS CALL IN THE PATIENTS WHO HAVE BEEN WAITING THE LONGEST FOR ADMISSION UNLESS OTHERWISE INSTRUCTED. DO THIS UNTIL ONE OF THE FOLLOWING TWO CONDITIONS OCCUR:
1. ALL PATIENTS ON THE SERVICE'S WAITING LIST HAVE BEEN PHONED.
2. THE NUMBER OF CONFIRMATIONS BY PHONE IS THE SAME AS THE # OF PATIENTS TO CALL IN (ON LINE 30).

Figure III-10 The 1 P.M. Decision Tables (Continued)

TABLE #2 -- FOR ASCS POTENTIAL CANCELLATION DECISION:
INCREASE IN AVAILABLE EMPTY BEDS EXPECTED TO OCCUR FOR ACUTE CARE
BASED ON THE TOTAL # OF DISCHARGES ALREADY OCCURRED BETWEEN 9 AM AND 1 PM

TOTAL # OF DISCHARGES IN HOSPITAL BETWEEN 9AM TO 1PM	SUN	MON	TUE	WED	THU	FRI	SAT	TOTAL # OF DISCHARGES IN HOSPITAL BETWEEN 9AM TO 1PM	SUN	MON	TUE	WED	THU	FRI	SAT
0	8	12	35	36	39	22	37	40	0	16	15	26	27	17	15
1	8	12	34	36	39	21	36	41	0	16	15	26	26	17	15
2	8	12	34	36	38	21	36	42	0	16	14	26	26	17	14
3	7	12	33	35	38	21	35	43	0	16	14	26	26	17	13
4	7	12	33	35	38	21	35	44	0	16	13	25	25	17	13
5	7	13	32	35	37	21	34	45	0	16	13	25	25	17	12
6	7	13	32	35	37	21	33	46	0	16	12	25	25	16	12
7	6	13	31	34	37	21	33	47	0	17	12	25	25	16	11
8	6	13	31	34	36	21	32	48	0	17	11	24	24	16	11
9	6	13	30	34	36	21	32	49	0	17	11	24	24	16	10
10	5	13	30	34	36	20	31	50	0	17	10	24	24	16	10
11	5	13	29	33	36	20	31	51	0	17	10	24	23	16	9
12	5	13	29	33	35	20	30	52	0	17	9	23	23	16	9
13	5	13	28	33	35	20	30	53	0	17	9	23	23	16	8
14	4	13	28	33	35	20	29	54	0	17	8	23	22	16	7
15	4	13	27	32	34	20	29	55	0	17	8	23	22	15	7
16	4	14	27	32	34	20	28	56	0	17	7	22	22	15	6
17	4	14	26	32	34	20	27	57	0	17	7	22	21	15	6
18	3	14	26	32	33	20	27	58	0	18	6	22	21	15	5
19	3	14	25	31	33	19	26	59	0	18	6	22	21	15	5
20	3	14	25	31	33	19	26	60	0	18	5	21	21	15	4
21	3	14	24	31	32	19	25	61	0	18	5	21	20	15	4
22	2	14	24	31	32	19	25	62	0	18	4	21	20	15	3
23	2	14	24	30	32	19	24	63	0	18	4	21	20	14	3
24	2	14	23	30	32	19	24	64	0	18	3	20	19	14	2
25	2	14	23	30	31	19	23	65	0	18	3	20	19	14	2
26	1	15	22	30	31	19	23	66	0	18	2	20	19	14	1
27	1	15	22	29	31	19	22	67	0	18	2	20	18	14	0
28	1	15	21	29	30	18	22	68	0	19	1	19	18	14	0
29	1	15	21	29	30	18	21	69	0	19	1	19	18	14	0
30	0	15	20	29	30	18	20	70	0	19	0	19	17	14	0
31	0	15	20	28	29	18	20	71	0	19	0	19	17	14	0
32	0	15	19	28	29	18	19	72	0	19	0	18	17	13	0
33	0	15	19	28	29	18	19	73	0	19	0	18	17	13	0
34	0	15	18	28	28	18	18	74	0	19	0	18	16	13	0
35	0	15	18	27	28	18	18	75	0	19	0	18	16	13	0
36	0	16	17	27	28	18	17	76	0	19	0	17	16	13	0
37	0	16	17	27	28	17	17	77	0	19	0	17	15	13	0
38	0	16	16	27	27	17	16	78	0	20	0	17	15	13	0
39	0	16	16	27	27	17	16	79	0	20	0	17	15	13	0

Figure III-11 Predicted Discharges Used in Conjunction with
Line 18 of the 1 P.M. Decision Tables (Figure III-10)

maintained by using call-in patients from any service after the other call-ins have been distributed across the services. Note that the CMAX call-in maximum (line 29) is 99 for the stream. As such, there is no practical constraint on the number of patients that can be called in via this stream. Discharges after 1 P.M. are also predicted in determining call-ins, Table 3 (Figure III-12) on line 23. Here discharges are predicted using the 50% point between the linear regression line and the minimum number of discharges. The more liberal point is chosen because we do not call in anyone if cancellations are predicted. Thus, the probability of not having enough beds is lower.

   c. The 3:30 P.M. Decision Tables

   Figure III-13 illustrates the 3:30 P.M. decision tables. These tables are essentially identical in format to the 1 P.M. tables. Of course in practice, the numbers will be different because of the elapsed time - 3:30 P.M. is the final decision point of the day. For the cancellation decision, line 18 uses Table 4 (Figure III-14). This table contains the 50% point of the difference between the regressed value and the lowest discharge value. The reasoning is that if a cancellation is indicated at this level on line 21, then the instructions of line 22 should be followed immediately to obtain the best possible estimate of discharges so that the actual discharges can be substituted for the estimated discharges before the final decision is made concerning cancellations.

   For the 3:30 P.M. call-in decisions, an estimate of the day's remaining discharges is entered on line 23 from Table 5 (Figure III-15). This table produces estimates based on the expected value predicted by the regression line alone (0% point). This results in the best estimate of the number of empty beds to expect due to discharges. Since call-ins should not occur unless the number of empty beds is above the CRA, errors in predicting discharges will tend to average out over a period of days.

   The delay of the last decision until 3:30 P.M. as far as the admission of surgical electives is concerned has to be made only if the 1:00 P.M. decision indicated that there is a potential problem. At 3:30 P.M., it is rather late in the day for this type of decision, but the last decision point is dictated by the discharge time of patients in the hospital. Perhaps, as hospital personnel see more clearly the negative consequences of late discharges, more attention will be paid to getting patients out early.

HOSPITAL 'XYZ'

TABLE #3 -- FOR ASCS CALLIN DECISION:
INCREASE IN AVAILABLE EMPTY BEDS EXPECTED TO OCCUR FOR ACUTE CARE
BASED ON THE TOTAL # OF DISCHARGES ALREADY OCCURRED BETWEEN 9 AM AND 1 PM

TOTAL # OF DISCHARGES IN HOSPITAL BETWEEN 9AM TO 1PM	SUN	MON	TUE	WED	THU	FRI	SAT
0	16	22	43	44	46	37	53
1	16	22	42	44	46	37	52
2	16	22	42	44	45	37	52
3	16	22	41	43	45	37	51
4	15	22	41	43	45	37	50
5	15	22	40	43	44	37	50
6	15	22	40	43	44	37	49
7	15	22	39	42	44	37	49
8	14	22	39	42	43	36	48
9	14	22	38	42	43	36	48
10	14	23	38	42	43	36	47
11	13	23	37	41	43	36	47
12	13	23	37	41	42	36	46
13	13	23	36	41	42	36	46
14	13	23	36	41	42	36	45
15	12	23	35	40	41	36	44
16	12	23	35	40	41	36	44
17	12	23	34	40	41	35	43
18	12	23	34	40	40	35	43
19	11	23	33	39	40	35	42
20	11	24	33	39	40	35	42
21	11	24	32	39	39	35	41
22	11	24	32	39	39	35	41
23	10	24	31	38	39	35	40
24	10	24	31	38	39	35	40
25	10	24	30	38	38	35	39
26	10	24	30	38	38	34	39
27	9	24	29	37	38	34	38
28	9	24	29	37	37	34	37
29	9	24	28	37	37	34	37
30	9	24	28	37	37	34	36
31	8	25	27	36	36	34	36
32	8	25	27	36	36	34	35
33	8	25	26	36	36	34	35
34	8	25	26	36	35	34	34
35	7	25	25	35	35	33	34
36	7	25	25	35	35	33	33
37	7	25	24	35	35	33	33
38	7	25	24	35	34	33	32
39	6	25	23	34	34	33	31

TOTAL # OF DISCHARGES IN HOSPITAL BETWEEN 9AM TO 1PM	SUN	MON	TUE	WED	THU	FRI	SAT
40	6	25	23	34	34	33	31
41	6	26	22	34	33	33	30
42	6	26	22	34	33	33	30
43	5	26	21	33	33	33	29
44	5	26	21	33	32	32	29
45	5	26	20	33	32	32	28
46	4	26	20	33	32	32	28
47	4	26	19	32	32	32	27
48	4	26	19	32	31	32	27
49	4	26	18	32	31	32	26
50	3	26	18	32	31	32	26
51	3	26	17	31	30	32	25
52	3	27	17	31	30	32	24
53	3	27	17	31	30	31	24
54	2	27	16	31	29	31	23
55	2	27	16	30	29	31	23
56	2	27	15	30	29	31	22
57	2	27	15	30	28	31	22
58	1	27	14	30	28	31	21
59	1	27	14	29	28	31	21
60	1	27	13	29	28	31	20
61	1	27	13	29	27	31	20
62	0	28	12	29	27	30	19
63	0	28	12	28	27	30	19
64	0	28	11	28	26	30	18
65	0	28	11	28	26	30	17
66	0	28	10	28	26	30	17
67	0	28	10	27	25	30	16
68	0	28	9	27	25	30	16
69	0	28	9	27	25	30	15
70	0	28	8	27	24	30	15
71	0	28	8	26	24	29	14
72	0	28	7	26	24	29	14
73	0	29	7	26	24	29	13
74	0	29	6	26	23	29	13
75	0	29	6	25	23	29	12
76	0	29	5	25	23	29	11
77	0	29	5	25	22	29	11
78	0	29	4	25	22	29	10
79	0	29	4	24	22	29	10

Figure III-12 Predicted Discharges Used in Conjunction with Line 23 of the 1 P.M. Decision Tables (Figure III-10)

TODAY'S DATE: _____   DAY OF THE WEEK: _____

PREPARED BY: _____

LINE#	ITEM	COL 1 MED_B	COL 2 SURG	COL 3 MED_A	COL 4 ONC_A	COL 5 NEU_NSU	COL 6 ONC_B	COL 7 FPR	COL 8 SWING	COL 9 ACUTE TOTALS
1	THE 1PM CALLIN MAXIMUMS (FROM PAGE #3, LINE #3)								XXXXXXX	XXXXXXX
2	ENTER THE # OF PATIENTS SUCCESSFULLY CALLED IN BETWEEN 1PM AND 3:30PM								XXXXXXX	XXXXXXX
3	THE 3:30PM CALLIN MAXIMUMS (LINE 1 - LINE 2)								XXXXXXX	XXXXXXX
4	UNIT CAPACITY	91	304	156	79	88	30	13	20	XXXXXXX
5	BEDS OUT OF SERVICE ON UNIT									XXXXXXX
6	SERVICEABLE BEDS ON UNIT (LINE 4 - LINE 5)									XXXXXXX
7	3:30PM CENSUS ON UNIT									XXXXXXX
8	# OF SERVICEABLE EMPTY BEDS ON UNIT AT 3:30PM (LINE 6 - LINE 7)	(+)	(+)	(+)	(+)	(+)	(+)	(+)	(+)	(=)
9	ENTER THE EXPECTED # OF TRANSFER REQUESTS FROM ACUTE TO ICU BETWEEN 3:30PM TODAY AND 9AM TOMORROW	XXXXXX	XXXXXX	XXXXXX	XXXXXX	XXXXXX	XXXXXX	XXXXXX	XXXXXX	XXXXXX
10	SUBTOTAL (LINE 8 + LINE 9)	XXXXXX	XXXXXX	XXXXXX	XXXXXX	XXXXXX	XXXXXX	XXXXXX	XXXXXX	XXXXXX
11	ENTER THE # OF PATIENTS SCHEDULED FOR ADMISSION TODAY BUT NOT YET ADMITTED	(+)	(+)	(+)	(+)	(+)	(+)	(+)	XXXXXX	(=)
12	ENTER THE # OF PATIENTS SUCCESSFULLY CALLED IN TODAY BUT NOT YET ADMITTED	(+)	(+)	(+)	(+)	(+)	(+)	(+)	XXXXXX	(=)
13	ENTER THE EXPECTED # OF TRANSFER REQUESTS FROM ICU TO ACUTE BETWEEN 3:30PM TODAY AND 9AM TOMORROW	XXXXXX	XXXXXX	XXXXXX	XXXXXX	XXXXXX	XXXXXX	XXXXXX	XXXXXX	XXXXXX
14	SUBTOTAL (LINE 11 + LINE 12 + LINE 13)	XXXXXX	XXXXXX	XXXXXX	XXXXXX	XXXXXX	XXXXXX	XXXXXX	XXXXXX	XXXXXX
15	EMPTY BED COUNT DIFFERENCE (LINE 10 - LINE 14)	XXXXXX	XXXXXX	XXXXXX	XXXXXX	XXXXXX	XXXXXX	XXXXXX	XXXXXX	XXXXXX

NOTE #1: "ACUTE TOTALS" IS USED IN THE DECISION TABLES TO DENOTE EITHER BEDS OR PATIENTS ASSOCIATED WITH THE SERVICES MED_A, MED_B, SURG, ONC_A, ONC_B, NEU_NSU, FPR AND THE SWING UNIT.

NOTE #2: WHEN "(+)" APPEARS IN THE BOX FORMED BY A COLUMN AND ROW, THEN ITS VALUE IS TO BE INCLUDED IN THE SUMMATION TO BE PLACED IN COLUMN #9 OF THE ROW. BOXES NOT CONTAINING "(+)" MUST BE OMITTED FROM THE ROW'S SUMMATION.

Figure III-13   The 3:30 P.M. Decision Tables

                                  3:30PM DECISION TABLE

TODAY'S DATE: _____   DAY OF THE WEEK: _____

PREPARED BY: _____

LINE#	ITEM	COL 1 MED_B	COL 2 SURB	COL 3 MED_A	COL 4 ONC_A	COL 5 NEU_NSU	COL 6 ONC_B	COL 7 FPR	COL 8 SWING	COL 9 ACUTE TOTALS
16	REENTER THE VALUE FROM LINE 15	XXXX	XXXX	XXXX	XXXX	XXXX	XXXX	XXXX	XXXX	
17	ENTER THE # OF PATIENTS DISCHARGED OR EXPIRED TODAY BETWEEN 9AM AND 3:30PM	(+)	(+)	(+)	(+)	(+)	(+)	(+)	(+)	(=)
18	FOR THE CANCELLATION DECISION: ENTER THE EXPECTED # OF EMPTY BEDS TO BECOME AVAILABLE BETWEEN 3:30PM TODAY AND 9AM TOMORROW DUE TO DISCHARGES (BASED ON LINE 17 AND TABLE #4)									
19	EXPECTED # OF SERVICEABLE EMPTY BEDS FOR THE CANCELLATION DECISION (LINE 16 + LINE 18)									
20	ENTER THE CANCELLATION ALLOWANCE (CAN) (FROM THE TABLE OF ASCS ALLOWANCES -- TABLE #1)									
21	THE EXPECTED # OF ASCS EMPTY BEDS FOR THE CANCELLATION DECISION (LINE 19 - LINE 20)									

| 22 | IF THE VALUE OF LINE 21 IS NEGATIVE, THEN IT REPRESENTS THE PRELIMINARY COUNT OF ADMISSIONS TO CANCEL FOR THOSE SCHEDULED PATIENTS NOT YET ADMITTED. IF THIS IS THE CASE, THEN:
  A. WARN THE ADMISSIONS OFFICE SUPERVISOR OF THE SITUATION SO THAT THE FOLLOWING PROCEDURES CAN BE INVOKED PRIOR TO CANCELLING:
    1. ASCERTAIN THE EXACT NUMBER OF ADDITIONAL EMPTY BEDS THAT WILL BE MADE AVAILABLE BY PATIENTS KNOWN TO BE DISCHARGED FROM ACUTE BEDS BETWEEN NOW AND 10PM. ENTER THE NUMBER HERE:
      _____
    2. IF THE NUMBER ASCERTAINED FOR ITEM 22.A.1 IS NOT GREATER THAN THE VALUE ON LINE 18, THEN LINE 21 REPRESENTS THE NUMBER OF PATIENTS TO CANCEL WITHOUT RECOMPUTATION.
    3. IF THE NUMBER ASCERTAINED FOR ITEM 22.A.1 IS GREATER THAN THE VALUE ON LINE 18, THEN REPLACE THE VALUE ON LINE 18 WITH THE ITEM 22.A.1 NUMBER AND RECOMPUTE LINE 19 AND LINE 21. IF THE RESULTING NUMBER OF ASCS EMPTY BEDS ON LINE 21 IS STILL NEGATIVE, THEN IT REPRESENTS THE FINAL NUMBER OF PATIENTS TO CANCEL.
  B. DISCONTINUE PROCESSING THE 3:30PM DECISION TABLES. DO NOT CALL IN ANY MORE PATIENTS. | | | | | | | | | |

LINE#	ITEM	COL 1 MED_B	COL 2 SURB	COL 3 MED_A	COL 4 ONC_A	COL 5 NEU_NSU	COL 6 ONC_B	COL 7 FPR	COL 8 SWING	COL 9 ACUTE TOTALS
23	FOR CALLIN DECISION: ENTER THE EXPECTED # OF EMPTY BEDS TO BECOME AVAILABLE BETWEEN 3:30PM TODAY AND 9AM TOMORROW DUE TO DISCHARGES (BASED ON LINE 17 AND TABLE #5)									
24	EXPECTED # OF SERVICEABLE EMPTY BEDS FOR CALLIN DECISION (LINE 16 + LINE 23)									
25	CENSUS REDUCTION ALLOWANCE (CRA) (FROM THE TABLE OF ASCS ALLOWANCES -- TABLE #1)									
26	# OF ASCS EMPTY BEDS AVAILABLE FOR 3:30PM CALLINS (LINE 24 - LINE 25)									

NOTE #1: "ACUTE TOTALS" IS USED IN THE DECISION TABLES TO DENOTE EITHER BEDS OR PATIENTS ASSOCIATED WITH THE SERVICES MED_A, MED_B, SURG, ONC_A, ONC_B, NEU_NSU, FPR AND THE SWING UNIT.

NOTE #2: WHEN "(+)" APPEARS IN THE BOX FORMED BY A COLUMN AND ROW, THEN ITS VALUE IS TO BE INCLUDED IN THE SUMMATION TO BE PLACED IN COLUMN #9 OF THE ROW. BOXES NOT CONTAINING "(+)" MUST BE OMITTED FROM THE ROW'S SUMMATION.

Figure III-13   The 3:30 P.M. Decision Tables (Continued)

3:30PM DECISION TABLE

TODAY'S DATE: _____   DAY OF THE WEEK: _____

PREPARED BY:
_____

PROCEDURE FOR CALCULATING # OF PATIENTS TO CALLIN:
1. PROCESS THE COLUMN FOR MEDB_#1 LINE 27 THRU LINE 31.
2. PROCESS THE COLUMN FOR MED_A LINE 27 THRU LINE 31.
3. PROCESS THE COLUMN FOR SURG LINE 27 THRU LINE 31.
4. PROCESS THE COLUMN FOR ONC_A LINE 27 THRU LINE 31.
5. PROCESS THE COLUMN FOR NEU_NSU LINE 27 THRU LINE 31.
6. PROCESS THE COLUMN FOR ONC_B LINE 27 THRU LINE 31.
6. PROCESS THE COLUMN FOR FPR LINE 27 THRU LINE 33.
8. PROCESS THE COLUMN FOR MEDB_#2 LINE 27 THRU LINE 31.

		COL 1	COL 2	COL 3	COL 4	COL 5	COL 6	COL 7	COL 8
LINE#	ITEM	MEDB_#1	SURG	MED_A	ONC_A	NEU_NSU	ONC_B	FPR	MEDB_#2
27	# OF ASCS EMPTY BEDS REMAINING FOR CALLINS (ENTER IN COL #1 THE VALUE FROM LINE 26, COL #9)								
28	ENTER THE SERVICE'S CALLIN WAITING LIST LENGTH AT 3:30PM (NOTE FOR MEDB_#2: TAKE INTO ACCOUNT THE # OF PATIENTS TO BE CALLED IN FOR MEDB_#1)								
29	ENTER THE 3:30PM CALLIN MAXIMUM FOR THE SERVICE (FROM LINE 3)								99
30	# OF PATIENTS TO CALLIN AT 3:30PM (TAKE THE MINIMUM OF LINE 27, LINE 28 AND LINE 29; IF THE RESULT IS NEGATIVE, THEN ENTER "0")								
31	# OF EMPTY BEDS REMAINING AFTER CALLINS (LINE 27 - LINE 30) (EXCEPT FOR FPR AND MEDB_#2, COPY THE VALUE CALCULATED TO LINE 27 IN THE NEXT COLUMN)								

IF THE COLUMN LAST PROCESSED ON LINE 31 WAS NOT FOR 'FPR' OR 'MEDB_#2', THEN CONTINUE WITH THE NEXT COLUMN ON LINE 27.

32	ENTER TODAY'S ADJUSTMENT FACTOR FOR MEDB_#2 CALLINS (FROM THE TABLE OF ASCS ALLOWANCES -- TABLE #1)	▨	▨	▨	▨	▨	▨		▨
33	ADJ5ST # OF EMPTY BEDS REMAINING FOR MEDB_#2 CALLINS (LINE 31 - LINE 32: PLACE THE VALUE HERE AND IN COLUMN #8 OF LINE 27).	▨	▨	▨	▨	▨	▨		▨

NOTE: THE PROCEDURE TO FOLLOW WHEN PHONING PATIENTS TO BE CALLED IN:
ALWAYS CALL IN THE PATIENTS WHO HAVE BEEN WAITING THE LONGEST FOR ADMISSION UNLESS OTHERWISE INSTRUCTED. DO THIS UNTIL ONE OF THE FOLLOWING TWO CONDITIONS OCCUR:
1. ALL PATIENTS ON THE SERVICE'S WAITING LIST HAVE BEEN PHONED.
2. THE NUMBER OF CONFIRMATIONS BY PHONE IS THE SAME AS THE # OF PATIENTS TO CALL IN (ON LINE 30).

Figure III-13   The 3:30 P.M. Decision Tables (Continued)

HOSPITAL 'XYZ'

TABLE #4 -- FOR ASCS CANCELLATION DECISION:
INCREASE IN AVAILABLE EMPTY BEDS EXPECTED TO OCCUR FOR ACUTE CARE
BASED ON THE TOTAL # OF DISCHARGES ALREADY OCCURRED BETWEEN 9 AM AND 3:30 PM

TOTAL # OF DISCHARGES IN HOSPITAL BETWEEN 9AM TO 3:30PM	SUN	MON	TUE	WED	THU	FRI	SAT
6	3	0	7	0	23	9	13
7	3	0	7	0	22	8	13
8	3	0	7	0	22	8	12
9	3	0	8	0	22	8	12
10	3	0	8	0	22	8	12
11	3	0	8	0	21	8	12
12	3	0	8	0	21	8	12
13	3	0	8	0	21	8	12
14	3	0	8	0	21	8	12
15	3	0	8	0	20	8	12
16	3	0	8	0	20	8	12
17	3	0	8	0	20	8	11
18	3	0	8	0	20	8	11
19	3	0	8	0	19	8	11
20	3	0	9	0	19	8	11
21	3	0	9	0	19	7	11
22	3	0	9	0	19	7	11
23	3	0	9	0	18	7	11
24	3	0	9	0	18	7	11
25	3	0	9	0	18	7	10
26	3	1	9	0	18	7	10
27	3	1	9	0	17	7	10
28	3	1	9	0	17	7	10
29	3	1	9	0	17	7	10
30	3	1	9	0	17	7	10
31	3	1	10	0	16	7	10
32	3	2	10	0	16	7	10
33	3	2	10	0	16	7	10
34	3	2	10	0	16	6	9
35	3	2	10	0	15	6	9
36	3	2	10	0	15	6	9
37	3	2	10	0	15	6	9
38	3	2	10	0	15	6	9
39	3	3	10	0	14	6	9
40	3	3	10	0	14	6	9
41	3	3	10	0	14	6	9
42	3	3	11	0	14	6	9
43	3	3	11	0	13	6	8
44	3	3	11	0	13	6	8
45	3	4	11	0	13	6	8
46	3	4	11	1	13	6	8
47	3	4	11	1	12	6	8
48	3	4	11	1	12	5	8
49	3	4	11	1	12	5	8
50	3	4	11	1	12	5	8

TOTAL # OF DISCHARGES IN HOSPITAL BETWEEN 9AM TO 3:30PM	SUN	MON	TUE	WED	THU	FRI	SAT
51	3	5	11	2	11	5	7
52	4	5	11	2	11	5	7
53	4	5	12	2	11	5	7
54	4	5	12	2	10	5	7
55	4	5	12	2	10	5	7
56	4	5	12	3	10	5	7
57	4	6	12	3	10	5	7
58	4	6	12	3	9	5	7
59	4	6	12	3	9	5	7
60	4	6	12	3	9	5	6
61	4	6	12	4	9	5	6
62	4	6	12	4	8	4	6
63	4	7	12	4	8	4	6
64	4	7	13	4	8	4	6
65	4	7	13	4	8	4	6
66	4	7	13	5	7	4	6
67	4	7	13	5	7	4	6
68	4	7	13	5	7	4	5
69	4	7	13	5	7	4	5
70	4	8	13	5	6	4	5
71	4	8	13	6	6	4	5
72	4	8	13	6	6	4	5
73	4	8	13	6	6	4	5
74	4	8	13	6	5	4	5
75	4	8	14	6	5	4	5
76	4	9	14	7	5	3	5
77	4	9	14	7	5	3	4
78	4	9	14	7	4	3	4
79	4	9	14	7	4	3	4
80	4	9	14	7	4	3	4
81	4	9	14	8	4	3	4
82	4	10	14	8	3	3	4
83	4	10	14	8	3	3	4
84	4	10	14	8	3	3	4
85	4	10	14	8	3	3	3
86	4	10	15	9	2	3	3
87	4	10	15	9	2	3	3
88	4	11	15	9	2	2	3
89	4	11	15	9	2	2	3
90	4	11	15	9	1	2	3
91	4	11	15	10	1	2	3
92	4	11	15	10	1	2	3
93	4	11	15	10	1	2	3
94	4	12	15	10	0	2	2
95	4	12	15	10	0	2	2

Figure III-14 Predicted Discharges Used in Conjunction with Line 18 of the 3:30 P.M. Decision Tables (Figure III-13)

HOSPITAL 'XYZ'

TABLE #5 -- FOR ASCS CALLIN DECISION:
INCREASE IN AVAILABLE EMPTY BEDS EXPECTED TO OCCUR FOR ACUTE CARE
BASED ON THE TOTAL # OF DISCHARGES ALREADY OCCURRED BETWEEN 9 AM AND 3:30 PM

TOTAL # OF DISCHARGES IN HOSPITAL BETWEEN 9AM TO 3:30PM	SUN	MON	TUE	WED	THU	FRI	SAT	TOTAL # OF DISCHARGES IN HOSPITAL BETWEEN 9AM TO 3:30PM	SUN	MON	TUE	WED	THU	FRI	SAT
6	9	11	13	10	33	26	25	51	10	18	17	19	22	23	19
7	9	11	13	10	33	26	25	52	10	18	18	19	21	23	19
8	9	11	14	10	33	26	24	53	10	19	18	19	21	23	19
9	9	11	14	10	32	26	24	54	10	19	18	19	21	23	19
10	9	12	14	10	32	26	24	55	10	19	18	19	21	23	19
11	9	12	14	11	32	26	24	56	10	19	18	20	20	22	19
12	9	12	14	11	32	26	24	57	10	19	18	20	20	22	19
13	9	12	14	11	31	26	24	58	10	19	18	20	20	22	19
14	9	12	14	11	31	26	24	59	10	20	18	20	20	22	18
15	9	12	14	11	31	25	24	60	10	20	18	20	19	22	18
16	9	13	14	12	31	25	23	61	10	20	18	21	19	22	18
17	9	13	14	12	30	25	23	62	10	20	18	21	19	22	18
18	9	13	14	12	30	25	23	63	10	20	19	21	19	22	18
19	9	13	15	12	30	25	23	64	10	20	19	21	18	22	18
20	9	13	15	12	30	25	23	65	10	21	19	21	18	22	18
21	9	13	15	13	29	25	23	66	10	21	19	22	18	22	18
22	9	14	15	13	29	25	23	67	10	21	19	22	18	22	18
23	9	14	15	13	29	25	23	68	10	21	19	22	17	22	17
24	9	14	15	13	29	25	23	69	10	21	19	22	17	22	17
25	9	14	15	13	28	25	22	70	10	21	19	22	17	21	17
26	9	14	15	14	28	25	22	71	10	21	19	23	17	21	17
27	9	14	15	14	28	25	22	72	10	22	19	23	16	21	17
28	9	15	15	14	28	25	22	73	10	22	19	23	16	21	17
29	9	15	15	14	27	24	22	74	10	22	20	23	16	21	17
30	9	15	16	14	27	24	22	75	10	22	20	23	16	21	17
31	9	15	16	15	27	24	22	76	10	22	20	24	15	21	16
32	9	15	16	15	27	24	22	77	10	22	20	24	15	21	16
33	9	15	16	15	26	24	22	78	10	23	20	24	15	21	16
34	9	16	16	15	26	24	21	79	10	23	20	24	15	21	16
35	9	16	16	15	26	24	21	80	10	23	20	24	14	21	16
36	9	16	16	16	26	24	21	81	10	23	20	25	14	21	16
37	9	16	16	16	25	24	21	82	10	23	20	25	14	21	16
38	9	16	16	16	25	24	21	83	10	23	20	25	14	21	16
39	9	16	16	16	25	24	21	84	10	24	20	25	13	20	16
40	9	16	16	16	24	24	21	85	10	24	21	25	13	20	15
41	9	17	17	17	24	24	21	86	10	24	21	26	13	20	15
42	9	17	17	17	24	24	20	87	10	24	21	26	12	20	15
43	9	17	17	17	24	23	20	88	10	24	21	26	12	20	15
44	9	17	17	17	23	23	20	89	10	24	21	26	12	20	15
45	9	17	17	17	23	23	20	90	10	25	21	26	12	20	15
46	9	17	17	18	23	23	20	91	10	25	21	27	11	20	15
47	9	18	17	18	23	23	20	92	10	25	21	27	11	20	15
48	10	18	17	18	22	23	20	93	10	25	21	27	11	20	15
49	10	18	17	18	22	23	20	94	10	25	21	27	11	20	14
50	10	18	17	18	22	23	20	95	10	25	21	27	10	20	14

Figure III-15 Predicted Discharges Used in Conjunction with Line 23 of the 3:30 P.M. Decision Tables (Figure III-13)

F.   Special Decision Rules for Holiday Periods

      In the United States, holidays occur, with the exception of
Christmas from 6 to 9 days per year. Generally, no elective
surgery is done on a holiday and results in the census of the
hospital dropping for as much as a two-week period using
conventional admissions systems. The ASCS system as previously
described is a steady-state system; i.e., a system that will
handle the admissions process under normal conditions. A holiday
is an abnormal situation where, in order to keep the census as
high as possible, the normal decision rules have to be modified.
      For purpose of illustration, suppose we have the following
Surgical Schedule:

	Sun	Mon	Tue	Wed	Thu	Fri	Sat
General Surgery	6	5	5	5	5	0	0

      Let us assume that the average length of stay (LOS) is 5.7
days. Now suppose Monday is a holiday on which no surgery is
done. Then, assuming that surgeries are admitted the day before
their operation, we would admit 0 instead of 6 patients on
Sunday.
      The first thing to do is to look at the waiting list
situation approximately one week before the holiday. The
following diagram may be helpful.

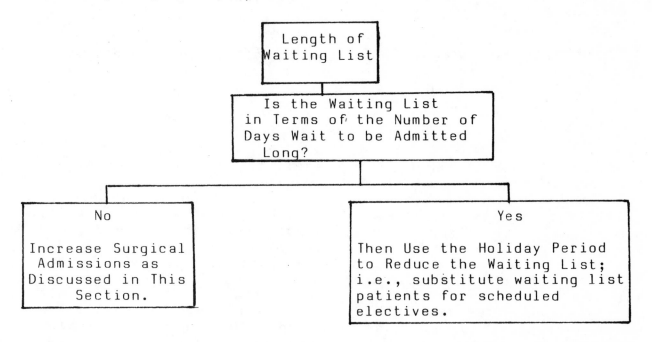

      If the waiting list is long (yes answer), then the number of
patients that will be called in will be automatically increased
via the call-in function. Thus holidays can be used to restore
the system balance without having to change schedules.

If the waiting list is not long (answer), then we can and should reschedule surgery as soon as possible. For example, if the holiday were on a Monday, then the six patients that were not admitted on Sunday should be scheduled as soon as possible after Sunday. A typical schedule would be:

Sun	Mon	Tue	Wed	Thu	Fri	Sat
0	7	7	7	5	0	0

The "ideal" schedule with respect to minimizing lost revenues would be:

Sun	Mon	Tue	Wed	Thu	Fri	Sat
0	11	5	5	5	0	0

Of course, under this schedule, we may be restricted by an operating room time constraint.

The lost patient days under the "typical" schedule would be:

	Lost Patient Days
Sunday	6
Monday	4
Tuesday	2
TOTAL	12

The lost patient days under the "ideal" schedule would be:

Sunday	6
Monday	0
TOTAL	6

Thus, the longer it takes to reschedule the patients, the higher the cost in terms of lost patient days.

If we decide to schedule additional patients, we have to "fool" the ASCS system because the call-in system, under normal procedures, will attempt to call in more patients on the day and days following the day that zero patients are scheduled (Sunday in the example). Thus on Sunday we must assume that all the allotted patients are scheduled when making call-in decisions. This will cause the call-in system to indicate call-ins as if all scheduled surgeries were to be admitted normally. Further, if we use the "typical" schedule as an example, we would, when making the call-in decisions, assume that the number of scheduled patients is as follows:

Sun	Mon	Tue	Wed	Thu	Fri	Sat
6	11	9	7	5	0	0

A rather unique situation occurs if the holiday comes toward the end of the week - Example: Thursday (Thanksgiving). In this case if it were to follow the "typical" schedule, we would reschedule as follows:

	Sun	Mon	Tue	Wed	Holiday Thurs	Fri	Sat
Week 1	6	5	5	0	7	0	0
Week 2	8	6	5	5	5	0	0

Lost Patient Days

Wednesday	5
Thursday	3
Friday	3
Saturday	3
Sunday	1
TOTAL	15

If no surgery were done on Friday either, then the lost days might be (over-schedule by two on Sunday, Monday, and by one on Tuesday):

Lost Patient Days

Wednesday	5
Thursday	5
Friday	5
Saturday	5
Sunday	3
Monday	1
Tuesday	0
TOTAL	24

Because of the high loss in patient days, we need to consider increased scheduling before the holiday. In some hospitals the discharge rate increases on Tuesday and Wednesday over the rate normally experienced. (Sometimes this occurs only on Wednesday.) This is probably due to patients desiring to be home for the holidays and/or because there will be someone home during the holidays to care for them. Also, on Monday the occupancy generally does not peak as it normally would, so there is excess capacity. Normally the excess capacity would be needed to prevent cancellations and turnaways on Wednesday and Thursday. If discharges are higher, then we should increase the schedule before the holiday in order to reduce lost patient days. The following is a possible schedule if we have increased discharges on Tuesday and Wednesday.

Sun	Mon	Tues	Wed	Thurs	Fri	Sat
6	7	7	0	6	0	0

The lost patient days would be:

Lost Patient Days

Monday	-2
Tuesday	-2
Wednesday	+5
Thursday	0
TOTAL	1

We do not need "to fool" the ASCS system for the increased scheduling before the holiday, but we do need to for all patients scheduled after the holiday.

CHAPTER IV

SYSTEM MONITORING AND DECISION NUMBER MAINTENANCE

A.   Introduction

The ASCS system is established using data on patient flows from the immediate past. These data are used to produce inputs for the simulator. In general, these inputs are:

1. Length of stay distributions for patients on each service and for each type of admission.

2. The patient arrival rates of each type of admission for each clinical service (unit).

3. The patient transfer rates between units.

4. Length of stay distributions for each of the patient transfer flows between units.

As long as the past and the future are inherently the same, then the decision rules do not need to be changed. However, the dynamics of hospital operations cause the flow of patients to change over time. Thus a system to monitor the basic assumption in establishing ASCS decision rules is needed so that resimulation can be performed to reestablish the decision numbers whenever it is appropriate to do so.

The principal objective of monitoring the ASCS is to detect problem situations as soon as they occur; i.e., whenever system inputs and/or outputs deviate from their intended operating ranges. To do this, the following input and output activity measures need to be recorded and periodically assessed by the ASCS management engineer:

1. Cancellations and Turnaways -- It is sufficient for the admissions department to record these system output measures in a journal when they occur.

2. Occupancy -- this is a system output measure which probably requires no futher recording and monitoring than is already being done by administration and the admissions department.

3. Waiting List Failures -- This is a system output measure and occurs whenever a patient on the waiting list gains admission as an emergency because his or her stay on the waiting list exceeded the "Maximum stay on Waiting List Policy" and he or she was not called in. Patients whose conditions deteriorate and are admitted as emergencies

without exceeding the Maximum Stay on Waiting List Policy are not Waiting List Failures. Waiting List Failures should be recorded in the same journal as cancellations and turnaways when they occur.

4. Waiting List Length -- This system input measure, though continuously maintained, should be regularly documented. If waiting list failures are a frequent problem, then the length of the waiting list should be recorded daily at the same time each day. If waiting list failures are not a significant problem, then it is sufficient to record the waiting list length on a weekly basis (designate one particular day of the week and time always to be used).

5. Waiting List Requests -- This system input measure need only be recorded if and when Waiting List Failures become a problem. If recorded, then the total number of requests for call-in admission that are placed on the waiting list each day should be recorded daily at the same time each day by the admissions department.

6. Patient Arrival Rates -- Each Patient Arrival Rate for each type of admission is a system input measure. For both scheduled and call-in admissions, retained copies of the daily ASCS Decision Rule computations are quite adequate for monitoring purposes. Emergencies (both through the emergency room and direct admits) are another matter and require that a daily record be maintained for the total number of emergency admissions to each major clinical division of the hospital. Definition of what constitutes a hospital's major clinical divisions depends to a large degree on hospital size and policy and is defined during implementation. Some hospitals may have four or five major clinical divisions, while a small community hospital may have only one or two. Because of the importance of this input activity measure, section B and section C of this chapter are devoted to further discussions of its recording and analysis.

B.   Changes in Arrival Rates

Of the simulator input data listed at the beginning of this chapter, the arrival rates have the most impact. Changes in patient mix, medical staff additions, and changes in hospital policies are the most common factors affecting the arrival rates over time horizons of six months to one year. Length of stay distributions and transfer rates also change, but experience indicates that their changes occur at much slower rates than patient arrival rate changes.

In order to be responsive to the hospital dynamics, it is necessary to monitor the patient flows so that all changes adversely affecting system performance may be detected. Some of the changes that occur are relatively easy for the admissions officer to detect and thus require no special detection procedures. For example, if the elective surgical demand started to increase, the system would respond by scheduling patients further into the future. Another example would be if the urgent (call-in) waiting list increases in length and results in urgent patients consistently failing to gain admission within the time horizon as specified by the hospital as an ASCS objective (waiting list failures).

But suppose the emergency arrival rate started to increase. The system would respond by cancelling surgery or by not having beds for emergent patients. However, both situations could also occur for other reasons such as clerical errors, improper scheduling during holiday periods, or the loss of bed capacity due to maintenance or construction. Thus we could need to know quickly if the emergency rates are increasing in order to determine the source of the problem. The assumption that is used in the simulator, which has been verified several times, is that emergency admissions are Poisson distributed with individual constant means for each day of the week.

C.   Control Charts as System Monitors

The Poisson assumption makes it relatively easy to establish control charts for system monitoring because the upper and lower control limits (confidence intervals) can be easily calculated or determined through table look-ups, and/or simple calculations.

Figure IV-1 is a typical daily control chart for direct admissions where the arrival rate is different for every day of the week. In this instance, the average daily arrival rates are:

Sun	Mon	Tue	Wed	Thur	Fri	Sat	TOT
0	8.2	7.3	7.6	6.7	7.5	3.8	39

The average daily rates change primarily because the number of physicians' offices that are open varies from day to day. The daily control limits are established using a cumulative Poisson table if the average is 20 and below. The normal approximation to the Poisson is used if the average is above 20.

These limits represent the extreme points still within range. Any points greater than the upper control limit or less than the lower control limit are said to be "out of control." Figure IV-2 gives the control limits for averages below 21. For averages above 20, an approximation based on the normal distribution is required for which the equations to use are:

$$\text{Upper Control Limit} = X + 1.96\sqrt{X} \tag{1}$$

$$\text{Lower Control Limit} = X - 1.96\sqrt{X} \tag{2}$$

Figure IV-3 is a control chart for admissions from the emergency room where the average daily rate is the same for each day of the week. This chart is easier to plot and use than that of Figure IV-1. If Figure IV-1 is found to be too difficult to use in the charting of direct admissions, then one may resort to a less technically correct, but easier to use method. This

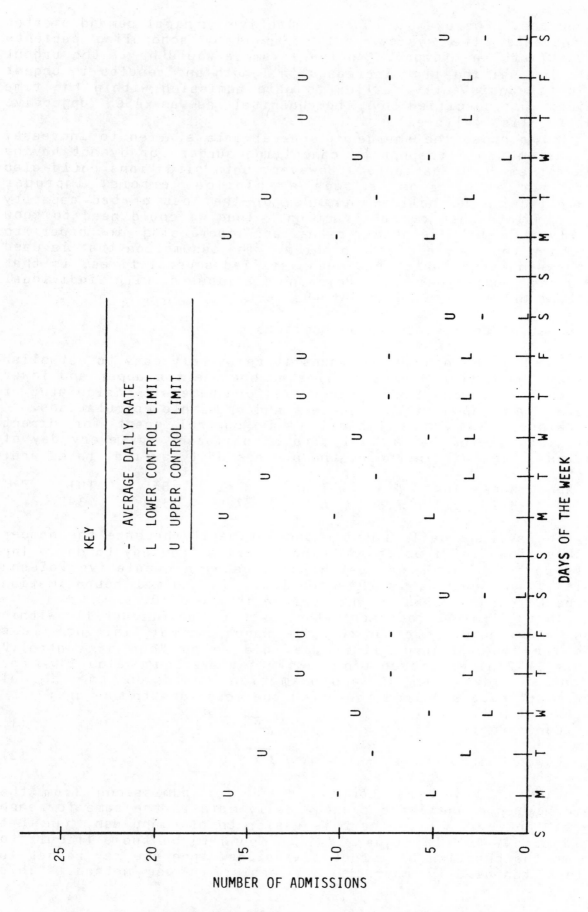

Figure IV-1 A Control Chart for Direct Emergent Admissions

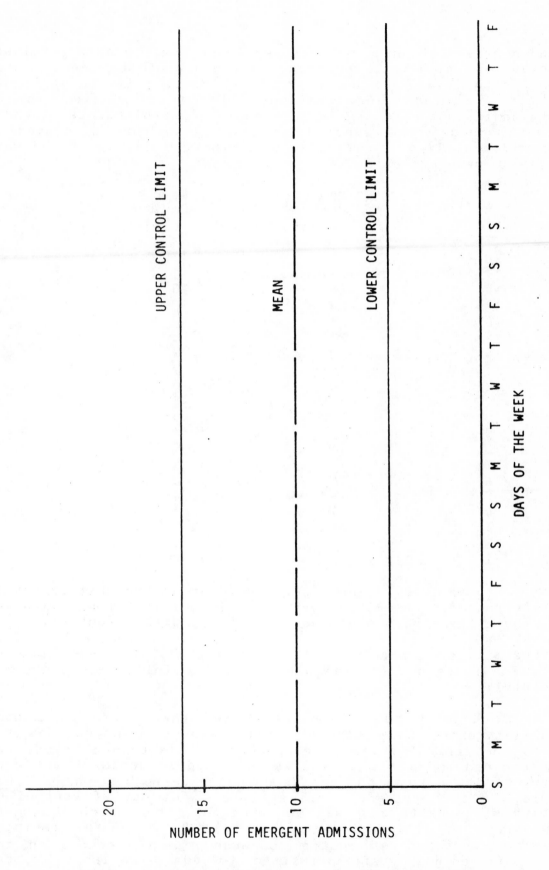

Figure IV-3 A Control Chart for Emergent Admissions From the Emergency Room

method consists of assuming that weekly arrival rates are Poisson
distributed. With this approach, we would plot the weekly rates
as in Figure IV-4. The Upper and Lower control limits of Figure
IV-4 were computed using equations (1) and (2) where X is the
weekly admissions rate. If we have out of control points, then it
will be necessary to revert to a chart like that displayed in
figure IV-1 or IV-3 in order to determine the day(s) of the week
for which problems exist.

X	Upper Control Limit	Lower Control Limit
20	28	12
19	27	11
18	25	10
17	24	10
16	23	9
15	22	8
14	20	7
13	19	7
12	18	6
11	17	5
10	15	5
9	14	4
8	13	3
7	11	2
6	10	2
5	9	1
4	7	1
3	6	0
2	4	0
1	2	0

Figure IV-2   The Upper and Lower Control Limits for
Daily Average Arrival Rates Less Than 21. Limit Values Represent
the Extreme Points of the Range Still Within Control.

Statistical control charts are easy to plot and easy to
read. For those not familar with them, the following points may
be helpful:

1. A point out of control means that there is a high
probability that some abnormal circumstance is occurring and
causing the arrival rates to change. If this unusual event can
be determined and if it is unlikely to happen again in the near
future, then the decision numbers do not have to be changed. For
example, if the emergency arrival rates went out of control on
the high side due to a school bus accident, then no changes need
to be made in the decision numbers.   But, if the emergent
admissions went out of control because of an increase in the
number of medical staff permitted to admit patients to the
hospital, then because emergent admissions are likely to continue
to be higher, the ASCS decision numbers should be changed.

2. Out of control occurs when admissions are either greater or lower than the control points, but out of control can also exist if there are a series of points (usually 5 or more consecutive) above or below the mean value. This indicates a trend which has a low probability of happening unless something significant has changed. For example, changes in the number of medical staff and the resultant change in the number of admissions are typically detected by this type of trend analysis. Figure IV-5 is an example of a process that was in control until the trend started occurring beginning with the second Tuesday. In the example there are six consecutive days where the admission rate was above the mean. On the sixth day (Sunday) the admission rate exceeded the upper control limit. This may or may not happen in all cases, but the probability of its happening is much greater than if no trend had been evident.

3. Out of control situations due to high admissions will, if the decision numbers are not corrected when appropriate, result in increased surgical cancellations and turnaways. For out of control situations on the low side, the ASCS system can partially react without modification because low emergent admissions will result in increased ability to call in urgent patients. A frequent experience occurs for hospitals that establish a policy of admitting urgent patients within a specified number of days: the emergency rates drop as the urgent admissions category gains acceptance. When and if this happens, the emergent rates will show trends and perhaps fall below the lower control limit. At the appropriate time, resimulation should occur because there will be some loss in occupancy by using decision numbers that are established based on higher emergency rates than actually exist.

D.   The Role of Historical Data Collection

Up to this point all discussion in this chapter has been concerned with the day-to-day maintenance procedures for the Decision Numbers. In addition to the data collection activities of the admissions department, a greater in-depth data collection process (Historical Data Collection) must also be carried out. This is the ongoing data collection process in which each patient's hosptial stay is tracked for service rendered by the various hospital services and the timing associated with service delivery. This is the same data collection process that occurs for the implementation process.

Via recent portions (6 to 12 months) of the Historical Data Collection, the various simulator inputs not included in the day-to-day monitoring by the admissions department can be accurately determined for any required resimulations. These inputs include the length of stay distributions and transfer rates between units. In addition, changes in the distribution of daily patient discharge times can be used to update any discharge prediction that is a part of the Decision Rules.

For more details on the Historical Data Collections see Chapter VII.

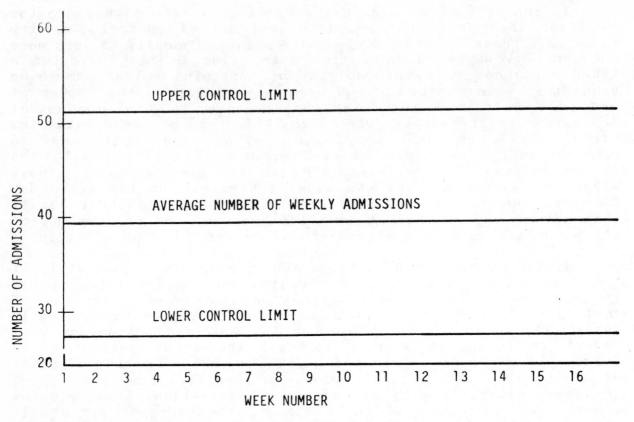

Figure IV-4 A Control Chart for Weekly Direct Emergent Admissions.

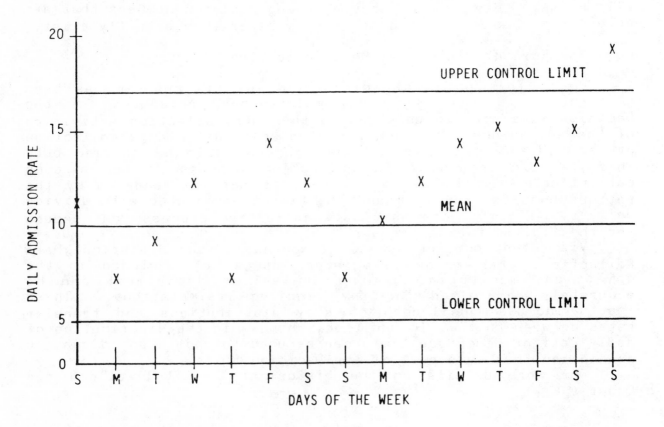

Figure IV-5 A Control Chart Showing a Trend

References:

1. Duncan A. Quality Control and Industrial Statistics, Richard D. Irwin, Inc., Fourth Edition, 1964.

CHAPTER V

BED-SIZING METHODOLOGY

A.   Introduction

When the first few ASCS admissions systems were installed,
it was observed that the maximum average occupancy predicted by
the simulator and the results achieved were substantially higher
than the professionally accepted occupancy figures used in
traditional planning processes at the time. Since higher average
occupancies were achievable, more patients could be served with
the same number of beds or the same number of patients could be
served with fewer beds. As a result, the ASCS simulator started
to be used as a planning tool to determine the potential maximum
average occupancy that hospitals and their units could achieve.

B.   Achievable Occupancies

As an example of these occupancies, Figure V-1 depicts a
series of curves that show the maximum achievable average
occupancies as a function of the number of beds, the percent of
elective patients that are advance-scheduled and the percentage
of patients that are emergency (assuming ASCS implementation)
(1).   Please note that the maximum average occupancy increases
as:

1. the number of beds increases,
2. the percent of advance-scheduled patients decreases, and
3. the percent of emergency admissions decreases.

Note also that the achievable maximum average occupancies
are greater than the 90% level that is widely accepted and
presently being used for planning purposes for medical/surgical
units.

The fact that predicted occupancies are higher than can be
obtained with any other presently documented admissions system
(2,3,4,5) has caused many potential users to be skeptical of the
realism of the ASCS and its simulation process. Countering this
skepticism, one has only to consult the results of Figures I-1
and I-2 to confirm the fact that the occupancies achieved via
the ASCS almost always equal or exceed the predictions.

C.   Evolution of the Methodology

From discussions with hospital planners, it became evident
that there was an urgent need for a technologically based
methodology that could readily predict occupancies, subject to
modifications for local conditions, yet be easily reproducible.
It was also apparent that such a methodology could be used prior
to an ASCS implementation in order to determine in advance
whether implementation would be worthwhile.

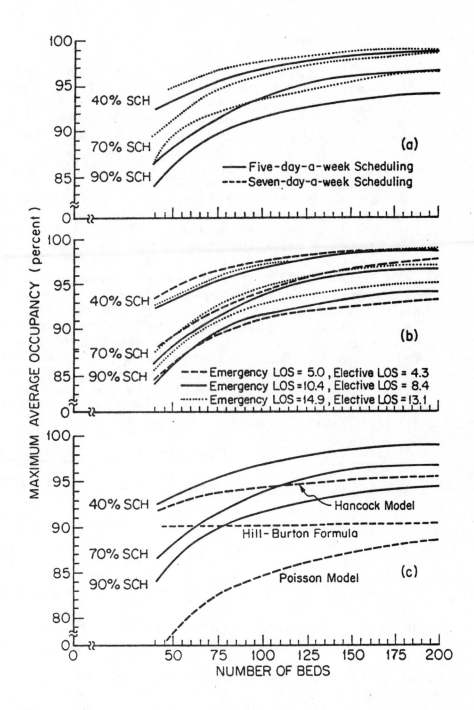

Figure V-1 Maximum Average Occupancy vs. Number of Beds for Different Percentages of Scheduled Arrivals and with 30, 50, and 66 Percent Emergency Arrivals

Reprinted with permission from Health Services Research, Vol. 13, No. 3, Fall 1978, p. 282. Published by the Hospital Research and Educational Trust, 840 North Lake Shore Drive, Chicago, Illinois 60611.

1. The Regression Equations

To meet these needs, the ASCS simulator was used in the development of prediction equations that could be used for a variety of purposes. By running the simulator hundreds of times according to an experimental design that assumed log-normal length of stay distributions, the necessary maximum average occupancy data were produced to be used in multiple regression analyses. The resultant regression equations had 20 to 25 terms and involved orthagonal transformations (6).

To date three sets of regression equations have been developed that predict occupancies for a large range of unit bed capacities (hereafter called bed sizes). Predictions by these equations are subject to the constraints of either: 1) a 1% maximum average cancellation rate for scheduled admissions and 1% maximum average turnaway rate for emergency admissions or 2) a 3% maximum average cancellation rate for scheduled admissions and 3% maximum average turnaway rate for emergency admissions. For all three equations, there is an assumption that no patient crossflow exists to or from other units for purposes of patient overflow or underflow. This implies that for the unit of prediction, an empty bed will be available for the scheduled or emergency arrival 97% of the time when a 3% equation is used and 99% of the time when the 1% equation is used. Figure V-2 illustrates the range and constraint levels for each of the equations.

	EQUATION # 1	EQUATION #2	EQUATION #3
RANGE OF BED SIZES	21 to 320	10 to 20	40 to 320
CANCELLATION AND TURNAWAY CONSTRAINTS	3%	3%	1%
APPLICABLE REFERENCES	6,7,8,9	6 and 8	6 and 8

FIGURE V-2   Range and Constraint Levels for
Three Regression Equations

The principal reason for having two equations for the 3 percent case is that desired accuracy cannot be maintained over the entire range of 10 to 320 beds using only one equation. For the one percent case, only one equation is used because 1% cancellations and 1% turnaways below the 40 bed level are deemed to be lower than necessary based upon actual practice.

2. Modification of the Methodology to Meet "Local" Conditions

Early use of the regression equations revealed that certain local conditions needed to be incorporated into the methodology in order to facilitate its use. Use of the methodology based on the equations alone produced reliable predictions, but assumed that weekly scheduled admission rates are constant throughout the year and that ample demand for elective call-in patients and emergency patients also exists throughout the year. This, however, is seldom the case because holidays, particularly Christmas and New Year's, impact most institutions to one degree or another by not scheduling surgery on these days. Since the methodology is intended for planning purposes, these factors have also been incorporated so that realistic average occupancy levels (over the course of an entire year) can be predicted as well. More specifically, the methodology provides for:

a. The number of holidays in the year (most hospitals do not have elective surgery on the holidays).

b. The characteristics of the Christmas/New Year season: i.e., the length of this particular holiday period and the estimated reduction in occupancy during the period that should be taken into account.

Hereafter, this local condition for holidays and the Christmas season will be referred to as the "Holiday and Christmas Effect."

A second local condition to be investigated and incorporated into the methodology involved the effect of weekend elective admissions. Because some third party reimbursers make exception to their payment policies for elective patients admitted on weekends, the methodology permits the user to specify whether or not weekend elective admissions are to be permitted (3% equations only).

The final local condition to be implemented resulted from analysis of one of the experimental design assumptions. The question the assumption raises is: "How different are the results if a local hospital's empirical length of stay distributions are used instead of the analytic log-normal distributions?" The analysis showed a reduction in maximum average occupancy that was significant at alpha = .05 for both with and without the weekend call-in local condition. Thus, difference equations were developed to handle the reduction (for 3% Large Unit Equation only).

D.   Use of the HP-41C for Processing the Methodology

To use the regression equations modified for local conditions with any degree of accuracy and reliability, a computational aid with alphanumeric input/output is essential. Although many computers are quite capable of performing the necessary calculations, their size, cost and complexity undermine the intended portability of the methodology. Fortunately, there is a hand-held calculator on the market with magnetic card reading capabilities and sufficient memory capacity to process the methodologies -- the Hewlett Packard HP-41C.

To date, the methodology has been fully implemented on the HP-41C. Reference 14 explains in detail the operation of the calculator for processing the methodology and can be obtained from the National Technical Information Service (NTIS) along with copies of the HP-41C magnetic card strips containing the programs and data.

1. Modes of Operation

By design, the equations are intended to predict the "Maximum average Occupancy" given that the values of the following variables are fixed:

a. Number of Beds

b. Percent Scheduled :

$$\frac{\text{The scheduled admission rate}}{\text{Total non-emergeny admission rate}} \times 100$$

c. Percent Emergency :

$$\frac{\text{The emergency admission rate}}{\text{The total admission rate}} \times 100$$

d. Average Elective (non-emergency) Length of Stay

e. Average Emergency Length of Stay

f. Variance in Length of Stays (of emergent and scheduled patients)

As an alternative application of the equations, it is also possible to determine the "Number of Beds Required at the point that Maximum Average Occupany is Achieved" given that the values of the following variables are fixed:

a. Average Daily Census

b. Percent Scheduled :

$$\frac{\text{The scheduled admission rate}}{\text{Total non-emergency admission rate}} \times 100$$

c. Percent Emergency :

$$\frac{\text{The emergency admission rate}}{\text{The total admission rate}} \times 100$$

d. Average Elective (non-emergency) Length of Stay

e. Average Emergency Length of Stay

f. Variance in Length of Stays

Briefly, this application involves a series of evaluations of the equations for maximum average occupancy. Initially the "Number of Beds" parameter is set to the values of the average daily census (ADC) parameter of this alternative application. By strategically increasing the "Number of Beds" parameter in each successive evaluation to a value equal to the ADC divided by the resulting maximum average occupancy of the previous evaluation, the resulting "Number of Beds" converges on the number of beds required at the point that maximum average occupancy is achieved for the given ADC.

Since it is desirable to use both of the above applications with and without the local conditions for holidays, four algorithms (called "Modes of Operation") have been established for each of the three equations. Before entering any of the parameter values, one of the four Modes of Operation in Figure V-3 must be selected for use:

MODE   MODE FUNCTION

a.   OCC   Maximum Average Occupancy

b.   OCHX   Maximum Average Occupancy with Holiday
              and Christmas Effects

c.   ALG   Algorithm for Bed Sizing Determination

d.   ALGHX   Algorithm for Bed Sizing Determination
              with Holiday and Christmas Effects

Figure V-3   Modes of Operation for the Bed Sizing
              Methodology using the HP-41C

2. HP-41C Methodology Messages and Responses

Because the HP-41C has only a limited character display window, prompting messages and messages indicating results may appear cryptic in their brevity to the novice. Figure V-4 is therefore presented as a key to each of the possible messages explaining the nature of the message and the appropriate user action when a response is required.

E.   Demonstration of the Methodology Using the HP-41C

To demonstrate the methodology four examples based on the HP-41C and the programs are presented. The figures accompanying the examples illustrate the printout that would occur from the user's interaction with the HP-41C if the calculator is connected to its thermographic printer.

1. Example #1

A unit has 187 beds. The % scheduled is 70% and the % emergencies is 33%. The length of stay is 6.2 days for elective patients and 8.2 for emergent patients. One percent cancellations and 1% turnaways are desired. What is the maximum average occupancy that is possible?

MESSAGE	EXPLANATION OF MESSAGE	USER RESPONSE
1% LU PGM	Message identifying the program as the '1% Large Unit Program'. Implies 1% turnaway and cancellation constraints for 40 <= BED SIZES <= 320.	NONE
3% LU PGM	Message identifying the program as the '3% Large Unit Program'. Implies 3% turnaway and cancellation constraints for 21 <= BED SIZES <= 320.	NONE
3% SU PGM	Message identifying the program as the '3% Small Unit Program'. Implies 3% turnaway and cancellation constraints for 10 <= BED SIZES <= 20.	NONE
WKEND 1=Y 0=N	Prompting message asking whether or not 'Weekend Elective Callins' are to be considered in processing.	Enter '1' for YES or '0' for NO.
ADC	For 'ALG' and 'ALGHX' modes, this is a prompting message requesting the the 'Average Daily Census' parameter be entered.	Enter a numerical value.
BEDS	For 'OCC' and 'OCHX' modes, this is a prompting message requesting that the 'Number of Beds' parameter be entered.	Enter a numerical value.
%SCH	Prompting message for 'Percent Scheduled' parameter.	Enter a value between 30.00 and 90.00 (between 0.00 and 100.00 for 3% SU PGM).
%EMG	Prompting message for 'Percent Emergency' parameter.	Enter a value between 30.00 and 90.00 (between 0.00 and 100.00 for 3% SU PGM).
ELL	Prompting message for 'Elective Length of Stay' parameter.	Enter a value between 4.50 and 15.00.
EML	Prompting message for 'Emergency Length of Stay' parameter.	Enter a value between 4.50 and 15.00.
VAR	Prompting message for 'Length of Stay Variance' parameter.	Enter a value between 9.00 and 135.00.
XMAS	Prompting message for 'Number of Days in Christmas Holiday Season' parameter.	Enter a numerical value.
%RDUC	Prompting message for '% Reduction' parameter; i.e., the % reduction in occupancy to occur during Christmas Holiday Season.	Enter a value between 0.00 and 100.00.
HDAY	Prompting message for 'Number of Holidays During Year Excluding Christmas Holiday Season' parameter.	Enter a numerical value.
OC=xx.xx%	Message presenting 'Percent Occupancy' result; xx.xx is a number.	NONE
BEDS =xxx.xx	For 'ALG' and 'ALGHX' modes, this is a message presenting the 'Number of Beds Required' result; xxx.xx is a number.	NONE
W/ DIF	Message indicating that the program results to follow are based on the use of the empirical length of stay distributions.	NONE

Figure V-4 Key to HP-41C Methodology Messages and Appropriate User Responses

```
               1% LU PGM
                 BEDS
          ---> 187.00
                 %SCH
          ---> 70.00
                 %EMG
          ---> 33.00
                 ELL
          ---> 6.20
                 EML
          ---> 8.20
                 VAR
          ---> 39.00
                 XMAS
          ---> 14.00
                 %RDUC
          ---> 30.00
                 HDAY
          ---> 6.00
               OC=93.13%
```

Figure V-5. The HP-41C Calculator Input and Output for Example
    #1

    In Figure V-5, the arrows indicate the data that were
entered as input. The length of stay (LOS) variance (VAR) was
set at 39 days. Normally this figure is not available, so Figure
V-6 was used to obtain an estimate of the LOS Variance. (6.20 +
8.20)/2 = 7.20. The closest LOS variance is 39.0.

Average of the Elective and Emergent Length of Stay	Estimate of LOS Variance
4.5	9.0
5.5	19.0
6.5	29.0
7.5	39.0
8.5	49.0
9.5	62.0
10.5	80.0
11.5	98.0
12.5	116.0
13.5	135.0

Figure V-6   Estimates of the LOS Variance Figures (12)
              as a Function of LOS

The XMAS Figure of 14.00 means that the Christmas Holiday Season will last 14 days and %RDUC (% Reduction) in occupancy during the Christmas Season was set at 30%. HDAY (Holidays) was 6.0 excluding the Christmas season.

The resulting predicted maximum average occupancy is 93.13%

2. Example #2

Suppose the unit is the same as in Example 1, but 3% cancellations and 3% turnaways are acceptable. Figure V-7 illustrates the input and the output for this HP-41C session.

```
        WKEND 1=Y 0=N
--->  1.00
        3% LU PGM
        BEDS
--->  187.00
        %SCH
--->  70.00
        %EMG
--->  33.00
        ELL
--->  6.20
        EML
--->  8.20
        VAR
--->  39.00
        XMAS
--->  14.00
        %RDUC
--->  30.00
        HDAY
--->  6.00
OC=95.71%
W/ DIF
OC=95.09%
```

Figure V-7   The HP-41C Input and Output for Example #2

The input of this session differs from that of Figure V-5 in that the first message "WKEND 1=Y 0=N" requests whether or not we can admit elective patients on the weekend. In this case we responded with a 1.00, which is a yes. The rest of the input is the same. Two occupancy figures are given. The first (95.71%) is based on the use of log-normal LOS distributions, which were also used in the Figure V-5 example. The second (95.09%) is an occupancy figure for which empirical length of stay distributions from five hospitals were used instead of the log-normal assumption (12). Please note that both occupancies are higher than those of Example 1. This is because a higher percentage of cancellations and turnaways is permitted (3% instead of 1%).

3. Example #3

Suppose we do not want elective admissions on the weekend because one of our third party reimbursers will not pay for the weekend days. What effect on occupancy would this have, assuming all other conditions were the same as in Example 2? The occupancy figures would be as follows:

OC=95.71%
W/ DIF
OC=93.34%

Here the log-normal occupancy does not change, but the actual LOS (W/ DIF) decreases. Although the maximum average occupancy does not change with the Log-normal LOS distributions, with actual distributions the ASCS admissions numbers change substantially. With no elective admissions on the weekend, the number of admissions on Sunday would have to be increased sharply in order to achieve the maximum average occupancy.

4. Example #4

A unit has an average daily census (ADC) of 150 patients. All other inputs are the same as in Example 2. We want to know the number of beds that would be needed.

```
        WKEND 1=Y  O=N
---> 1.00
        3% LU PGM
        ADC
--->150.00
        %SCH
---> 70.00
        %EMG
---> 33.00
        ELL
---> 6.20
        EML
---> 8.20
        VAR
---> 39.00
        XMAS
---> 14.00
        %RDUC
---> 30.00
        HDAY
---> 6.00
OC=95.28%
BEDS =157.43
W/ DIF
BEDS =158.45
OC=94.66%
```

Figure V-8   The Computer Output for Example 4

Figure V-8 contains the output. The results show that 158
beds (157.43) are needed with log-normal LOS distributions and
159 (158.45) beds with actual LOS distributions. This mode,
where the ADC is entered rather than the number of beds, is much
more useful to planners because they usually have an ADC and want
to know the number of beds needed.

F.   Input Ranges and Accuracy Considerations

The programs are designed to be "user friendly." They are
designed to indicate to the user whenever the user inputs a
parameter value that exceeds the limitation of the data ranges.
Figure V-9 contains the input ranges. If any of the above
limitations is exceeded, the calculator responds with an error
message so that the user will know that extrapolation is
occurring. The programs will still run and in many cases will
still provide good estimates, but the extent of error is unknown.

	Number of Beds	% Scheduled	% Emergent	LOS	LOS Variance
1% Large Unit Program	40-320	30%-90%	30%-90%	4.5-15.0	9-135
3% Large Unit Program	21-320	30%-90%	30%-90%	4.5-15.0	9-135
3% Small Unit Program	10-20	0%-100%	0%-100%	4.5-13.5	9-135

Figure V-9   The Data Input Ranges for the
Regression Equations

The prediction error, i.e., the error between the actual
simulated data points and the regression equations is contained
in Figure V-10.

1. 1% Large Unit Program --   Less than 1% occupancy error
                              with 90% confidence

2. 3% Large Unit Program --   Less than 1% occupancy error
                              with 95% confidence for the
                              log normal LOS distributions

3. 3% Small Unit Program --   Less than 2% occupancy error
                              with 95% confidence

Figure V-10 The Prediction Acccuracy of the Regression Equations
as Compared to the Simulated Data Points

G. Economic Calculations to Determine the Value of an
    Installation of the ASCS System.

    The use of these analyses is recommended as part of the
process of deciding whether or not to introduce the ASCS system.
The rationale is that, in general, one should not implement the
ASCS system unless it can be made clear in advance that the
advantages (savings) exceed the costs. The cost of
implementation should be recoverable within one year following
ASCS start-up. Two situations occur:

        1. Where the hospital, if it can increase occupancy, has
           sufficient demand.

        2. Where the ADC cannot be increased, the hospital
           desires to reduce the bed capacity to supply the
           service at minimum cost.

    For the first case, the hospital can increase its revenues
if the ASCS installation results in increased occupancy. The
calculations are as follows:

$$R = .01 \ (O_1 - O_2) \ B \times 365 \times D \qquad\qquad (1)$$

              Where:

              O_1 is the occupancy before installation of
                   the ASCS in %
              O_2 is the occupancy predicted for ASCS using
                   the bed-sizing equations in %
              B is the number of beds involved
              D is the Daily revenue rate/bed where

              $$D = \frac{Total \ Inpatient \ Budget}{365 \times B} \qquad\qquad (2)$$

              R is the increase in revenue in dollars

    For example, suppose a hospital has 250 beds and an
inpatient budget of $36,000,000. The present occupancy is 85%
and the predicted occupancy is 90.5%. Then using equation (2),

        $$D = \frac{\$36,000,000}{365 \times 250} = \$394.52$$

and using equation (1),

        $$R = .01 \ (90.5 - 85) \ 250 \times 365 \times \$394.52$$
        $$= \$1,979,997.25$$

which is the predicted annual savings. Suppose the total cost to install the ASCS system is $45,000. Then:

$$\frac{\$1,979,997}{\$45,000} = 44.0 \text{ is the annual rate of return}$$

of one year's savings vs. costs. Therefore on the basis of increased revenues, the installation is easily justified!

For the second case, the hospital cannot increase its demand, but wants to reduce its costs. If the hospital has 250 beds as in case 1, then:

$$250 \times 85\% \times .01 = 212.5 \text{ which is the ADC.}$$

Now suppose we use the bed-sizing algorithm and find that 234 beds are needed for an ADC of 212.5 and the other local conditions (% scheduled, % emergent, Christmas season, etc.). The calculations to determine the predicted cost savings are as follows:

$$CS = (B_1 - B_2) \times 365 \times D \times V \times .80 \qquad (3)$$
$$CS = \text{Cost Savings in dollars}$$

Where: B_1 = the original bed complement
B_2 = the predicted beds needed using the bed sizing algorithms
D = the daily revenue rate/bed as defined previously. The figures used are from case 1.
V = the estimated variable cost/bed over the time horizon of one year. The fraction of the total inpatient budget that is variable can, in the authors experience, be easily estimated by the chief financial officer provided that it is made clear that the variable costs are those costs that can be changed over a relatively long time horizon (at least one year). For our Case 2 example, a typical value of .60 has been used.
.80 = a factor that is intended to compensate for the fact that only 80% of the cost reductions will be realized because sometimes staffs cannot be reduced by a fraction of an FTE.

By Substituting in Equation (3), we get:

$$CS = (250-234) \times 365 \times \$394.52 \times .60 \times .80$$
$$= \$1,105,918.46$$

Please note that the cost savings, although substantial, are lower than the increases in revenues of case 1. The rate of return for one year's savings, assuming a cost of implementation of $45,000, would be $1,105,918.46/$45,000 = 25. Again the implementation is easily justified.

H.   Use of the Methodology to Investigate Changes in Hospital Policy

Suppose a hospital wants to use its excess capacity to be able to advance-schedule more patients. For example, a unit has 200 beds, 50% advance-scheduled, 30% emergency, an average LOS of 6.5 days, an LOS variance of 39, a 14-day Christmas season that results in a 30% reduction in occupancy, 6 holidays other than the Christmas season and an overall occupancy of 85%. What can be done to increase the number of advance-scheduled patients using the extra capacity that would result from installation of the ASCS?

The solution is obtained by using the bed-sizing methodology but increasing the % scheduled until the number of beds indicated equals the present occupancy. If we input the maximum % scheduled that the basic data will permit (90%), we will need 187 beds. Thus we can increase the scheduled electives from 50% to 90% and still have thirteen beds excess capacity.

It is frequently of interest to be able to talk in terms of the number of patients that can be advance-scheduled per week rather than the corresponding percentage of elective patients. The calculations to do this are as follows:

$$P = \frac{7 \times ADC}{LOS} \times (1.0 - (.01 \times E)) \times (.01 \times S) \qquad (4)$$

where:

   P = the patients/week scheduled.
   E = the % emergent.
   S = the % scheduled.
   ADC = the average daily census.
   LOS = the average length of stay.

For the 50% advanced scheduled case in the problem:

$$P = \frac{7 \times 170}{6.5} \times (1.0 - (.01 \times 30)) \times (.01 \times 50) = 64.08$$

and for the 90% advanced scheduled case in the problem:

$$P = \frac{7 \times 170}{6.5} \times (1.0 - (.01 \times 30)) \times (.01 \times 90) - 115.34$$

The difference between the two results, 115.34 - 64.08 = 51.26 implies that 51 additional patients can be advance-scheduled per week through the use of the ASCS and still have the thirteen-bed excess capacity calculated earlier.

I. References

1. Hancock, W.; Magerlein, D.; Storer, R.; and Martin, J. "Parameters Affecting Hospital Occupancy and Implications for Facility Sizing, Health Sciences Research, Vol. 13, No. 3, Fall 1978, p. 276-289.

2. Robinson, G., Wing, P.; and Davis, L. (1968) "Computer Simulation of Hospital Patient Scheduling Systems." Health Services Research, 3, p. 130-141.

3. Schonick, W. (1972), Understanding the Nature of Random Fluctuations of Hospital Daily Census", Medical Care, 10, p. 118-142.

4. Schonick, W. (1970) "A Stochastic Model for Occupancy-Related Random Variables in General-Acute Hospitals," Journal of the American Statistical Assoc., 65, p. 1474-1499.

5. Young, J. (1962) " A Queueing Theory Approach to the Control of Hospital Inpatient Census," Ph.D. dissertation, The Johns Hopkins University, School of Engineering Sciences.

6. Magerlein, M. "Maximum Average Occupancy and the Resultant Bed Size of Inpatient Hospital Units," Ph.D. Thesis, The University of Michigan, 1978.

7. Magerlein, D. and Hancock, W. "The Use of Simulation in the Determination of Maximum Occupancy for Hospital Facilities," Chapter 10 in Current Issues in Simulation, Academic Press, 1979, p. 137-163.

8. Gonzales-Pinon, M. and Hancock, W. "Use of the HP-41C Program for Calculating Hospital Maximum Average Occupancy and the Resultant Bed Size," unpublished, Bureau of Hospital Administration, The University of Michigan, 1979.

9. Hancock, W.; Martin, J.; and Storer, R. "Simulation-Based Occupancy Recommendations for Adult Medical/Surgical Units Using Admissions Scheduling Systems," Inquiry, Vol. XV, No. 1, 1978, p. 25-32.

10. Magerlein, D. and Hancock, W. "The Use of Simulation in the Determination of Maximum Occupancy for Hospital Facilities," Chapter 10 in Current Issues in Computer Simulation, N. Adam and A. Dogramaci, eds., Academic Press, 1979.

11. Goodale, N.; Hancock, W.; and Magerlein, D. "The Effect on Hospital Occupancy of Reducing Turnaways and Cancellations," Bureau of Hospital Administration, The University of Michigan, Report No. 79-2.

12. Langer, S.; Hancock, W.; and Luttman, R. "Users' Manual for
    the HP41-C Calculator for Use with Program to Calculate
    Maximum Average Occupancy and the Resultant Bed Size Using
    Empirical LOS Distributions With and Without Weekend
    Electives," Bureau of Hospital Administration, The
    University of Michigan, October 1980, Report 80-2.

13. Hancock, W.; Luttman, R.; Walter, P.; and Langer, S.
    "Comparison of Maximum Average Occupancy of Hospital Units
    Using Log-Normal and Empirical Length of Stay
    Distributions Where Elective Patients Are and Are Not
    Admitted on Weekends, Department of Hospital
    Administration, The University of Michigan, October 1980,
    Report No. 80-3.

14. Langer, B.; Hancock, W.; and Pinon, M. "Use of the HP41-C
    Program for Calculating Hospital Maximum Average Occupancy
    and the Resultant Bed Size with Difference Equations so
    that Log Normal or Empirical Distributions Can Be Used,"
    Report No. 80-3, Bureau of Hospital Administration,
    University of Michigan, October 1980.

CHAPTER VI

THE IMPLEMENTATION PROCESS

A.   The Initial Work

Because of the costs involved (both money and time) in
implementing the ASCS system, several preliminary steps are
usually taken to make sure that the ASCS will be an effective
system solution for some of the hospital's problems and that
there are adequate data available to provide the necessary input
to the ASCS simulator. These steps are:

1. Cost Effectiveness

An analysis is performed to determine the cost effectiveness
of installing the system.   The bed-sizing equations that are
presented in Chapter V are used for this purpose. Usually this
analysis involves the proper sizing of each unit of the hospital
as well as the sizing of groups of units where off-unit patients
are permitted. These results are generally presented in written
form to the appropriate hospital personnel and sometimes to
members of the medical staffs.

2. Data Adequacy

A determination is made of the adequacy of the data bases
necessary to develop the decision numbers/rules via the ASCS
Simulator. Chapter VI contains a discussion of the data needed
and the rationale. Unfortunately, the hospital data normally
available at the outset of an investigation are not sufficient to
use in the simulator without first establishing additional
special data collection procedures. The most frequent problems
encountered are:

   a. The hospital collects the necessary data, but purges
      its files once the patient bill is paid. Since six
      months of patient flow data is necessary to properly
      establish the length of stay distributions and the
      daily arrival rates, policies of file purging must be
      changed so that the six months of data can be
      accumulated.

   b. The medical abstracts office is not properly
      coordinated with the hospital, so that different
      terms are used and/or the proper data are not
      abstracted. For example:

1) Some abstracting offices decide on whether or not a patient is emergent as a function of diagnosis and pay little attention to how the patient was actually admitted or to the type of admission already determined by the admissions department.

2) The most common shortcoming of abstracting services is that they do not enable the patient's stay in the hospital to be "tracked" with respect to sequence and/or numbers of days on each of the services. When this occurs, either assumptions have to be made regarding the clinical services a patient used as a function of other information contained in the abstract or special data collections need to be established. This is not serious for a community hospital because of the relatively small number of clinical units to which a patient can be transferred, but it can cause substantial errors with teaching hospitals because of the number of transfers between specialized clinical units. In this case, special studies are necessary to get the proper data in order to obtain the length of stay distributions, the ADC of the various units and the transfer rates between units.

3) Some abstracting systems are designed to collect patient data according to the patient's specific functional care needs. In many instances there is no one-to-one mapping of these functional need categories to the hospital's established service categories. When this occurs, a large amount of time is required to create a realistic mapping based on additonal abstract fields such as age, diagnosis, physician codes, and surgical procedure codes. In addition further data collection and analysis are required to corroborate the mapping assumptions.

4) Many hospitals have policies concerning time of discharges, but practically none have the admini-strative systems to enforce the policies. Thus, discharges frequently occur until the late af-ternoon or early evening. Figure VI-1 is a his-togram of discharge time from a hospital with an 11 A.M. policy. To further complicate matters, the distribution of discharge times is day-of-the-week specific. Thus, if the abstract process does not record discharge time, a special data collection for a period of three or more months is necessary to obtain the necessary discharge time distributions.

DISTRIBUTION OF DISCHARGES THROUGHOUT THE DAY
(FOR MONDAY)

```
TIME_DIS              EACH X =   5 POINTS   COUNT = 1203    MEAN =   1359.3308     STD. DEV. =    413.5396

       FREQUENCY       PERCENTAGE                           25.0      75.0      125.0     175.0     225.0     275.0     325.0     375.0
       INT.  CUM.      INT.   CUM.                      0.0      50.0      100.0     150.0     200.0     250.0     300.0     350.0     400.0
                                        INTERVAL        +----+----+----+----+----+----+----+----+----+----+----+----+----+----+----+----+
          5      5     0.4    0.4    [12:00AM -  1:00AM) +X
          2      7     0.2    0.6    [ 1:00AM -  2:00AM) +X
          3     10     0.2    0.8    [ 2:00AM -  3:00AM) +X
          2     12     0.2    1.0    [ 3:00AM -  4:00AM) +X
          0     12     0.0    1.0    [ 4:00AM -  5:00AM) +
          3     15     0.2    1.2    [ 5:00AM -  6:00AM) +X
          1     16     0.1    1.3    [ 6:00AM -  7:00AM) +X
          3     19     0.2    1.6    [ 7:00AM -  8:00AM) +X
         12     31     1.0    2.6    [ 8:00AM -  9:00AM) +XXX
        100    131     8.3   10.9    [ 9:00AM - 10:00AM) +XXXXXXXXXXXXXXXXXXXX
        208    339    17.3   28.2    [10:00AM - 11:00AM) +XXXXXXXXXXXXXXXXXXXXXXXXXXXXXXXXXXXXXXXXXX
        192    531    16.0   44.1    [11:00AM - 12:00PM) +XXXXXXXXXXXXXXXXXXXXXXXXXXXXXXXXXXXXXXXX
        110    641     9.1   53.3    [12:00PM -  1:00PM) +XXXXXXXXXXXXXXXXXXXXXX
         81    722     6.7   60.0    [ 1:00PM -  2:00PM) +XXXXXXXXXXXXXXXXX
         92    814     7.6   67.7    [ 2:00PM -  3:00PM) +XXXXXXXXXXXXXXXXXX
         91    905     7.6   75.2    [ 3:00PM -  4:00PM) +XXXXXXXXXXXXXXXXXX
         70    975     5.8   81.0    [ 4:00PM -  5:00PM) +XXXXXXXXXXXXXX
         21    996     1.7   82.8    [ 5:00PM -  6:00PM) +XXXXX
         39   1035     3.2   86.0    [ 6:00PM -  7:00PM) +XXXXXXXX
         32   1067     2.7   88.7    [ 7:00PM -  8:00PM) +XXXXXXX
         32   1099     2.7   91.4    [ 8:00PM -  9:00PM) +XXXXXXX
         19   1118     1.6   92.9    [ 9:00PM - 10:00PM) +XXXX
         39   1157     3.2   96.2    [10:00PM - 11:00PM) +XXXXXXXX
         46   1203     3.8  100.0    [11:00PM - 12:00AM) +XXXXXXXXXX
                                                        +----+----+----+----+----+----+----+----+----+----+----+----+----+----+----+----+
                                                    0.0      50.0      100.0     150.0     200.0     250.0     300.0     350.0     400.0
                                                         25.0      75.0      125.0     175.0     225.0     275.0     325.0     375.0
```

Figure VI-1 The Distribution of Discharge Times from a Typical
Teaching Hospital

3. Liaison Arrangements

Compared to the administrative technologies that hospital administrations typically encounter, the ASCS technology is complex. This is also true for the management engineering group of the hospital. Thus a certain amount of education must occur so that the hospital can maintain the system once it is implemented. Part of the contractual arrangement is that a management engineer with expertise in computers be assigned to the project part-time in order to learn first-hand the necessary steps to implement and maintain the system. This education process is very helpful because the management engineer can coordinate the collection of data, can answer questions posed by hospital personnel, and can help in the training of the admissions personnel in the use of the decision rules.

B. The Use of the ASCS Simulator

1. Inpatient Flow Policies

After the necessary data is collected a pictorial summary of the hospital inpatient flow process is developed. Figure VI-2 is an example of a portion of the model which is part of the preliminary data analysis. This model is a vector diagram of the inpatient flows into and out of the unit as recorded in the patient flow data. A diagram like Figure VI-2 is displayed for every clinical unit within the hospital whose admissions are going to be controlled by the ASCS system.

This pictorial summary is then used to help the administration decide the most appropriate administrative policies, such as:

      a. The permissible cross flow of patients between units. For example, if an emergency medical patient needs to be admitted and there are no beds on the patient's intended medical service, what off-service units can admit the patient and what is the order of preference for these off-service units?

      b. If patients can be admitted to off-service units, is there any limit to the number of patients that the off-service unit can accommodate?

Most hospitals have implicit policies concerning the above, but different groups may perceive the policies differently. Many of the policies may contradict one another as well as be inconsistent with the overall needs of the hospital. Several meetings of all parties involved are often required to arrive at a consensus on the specific policies to be used. On occasion, it is necessary for a hospital to revise its current policies in advance of the ASCS start-up date because of the major shift in philosophy that will be required upon ASCS start-up.

TYPE OF ADMISSION table (left):

TYPE OF ADMISSION	ARRIVAL RATES DAILY	WEEKLY	MEAN LOS	AVG. DAILY CENSUS
EMERGENCY	2.948	20.635	11.52	33.971
CALL-IN	0.632	4.425	15.24	9.639
SURG_SCHED	4.113	28.791	8.86	36.423
GYN_SCHED	1.496	10.470	4.22	6.312

SURGERY UNIT (SURG) | 3 |

OVERALL BREAKDOWN BY SUB-UNIT

SUB-UNIT	ARRIVAL RATES DAILY	WEEKLY	MEAN LOS	AVG. DAILY CENSUS
SURG1	2.103	14.723	7.64	16.062
SURG2	1.191	8.335	8.74	10.404
SURG3	0.749	5.242	6.45	4.928
SURG4	0.574	4.015	6.08	3.490
SURG5	0.685	4.796	13.93	9.544
SURG6	0.829	5.800	5.06	4.191
SURG7	2.071	14.500	14.28	29.573
SURG8	2.183	15.280	8.88	19.376
TOTAL	10.384	72.691	9.39	97.468

TRANSFERS table (right):

ARRIVAL RATES DAILY	WEEKLY	MEAN LOS	AVG. DAILY CENSUS	TRANSFERS FROM
0.605	4.238	11.29	6.036	ICU_CCU
0.223	1.562	10.00	2.231	MED
0.367	2.570	5.60	2.056	OBS

DISCHARGE & TRANSFER BREAKDOWN

DESTINATION	AVERAGE RATES DAILY	WEEKLY	% OF TOTAL
DISCHARGE	9.114	63.800	87.77
ICU_CCU	0.574	4.015	5.52
OBS	0.489	3.426	4.71
MED	0.207	1.450	1.99

CAP NOW = 110 | SIZED CAP =

Figure VI-2   A Typical Vector Diagram for a Hospital Unit

2. Determination of the First and Last Decision Points

Prior to construction of the simulation model, it is necessary to determine the first and final Decision Point in the day. The first decision point is normally set at 9 A.M. prior to the admission of the day's elective patients. It marks the starting point of the ASCS day. The final one is the time at which the admissions office will make their last determination for the day (aided by the ASCS) of the numbers of scheduled admissions that must be cancelled and rescheduled or the numbers of patients to call in from the waiting lists. Selection of the final decision point depends on two factors:

    a. Ideally, an average of 80% of the day's discharges should occur between the first and final decision points. Histograms similar to that of Figure VI-1 are very helpful in this respect.

    b. For those hospitals that might require a late afternoon final decision point because of their late discharges, some consideration must be given to the problem this will cause for the late in the day call-in of waiting list patients. The later it is, the more problems it will cause for both the patients and the hospital's ancillary services.

The reason the determination of these decision points must be made prior to model construction is that the model's emergency arrival rates have to be determined according to the number of emergencies that arrive between the first and final decision points, and the number of emergencies that arrive after the final decision point but before the first decision point of the next day.

3. The Building of the Simulator Model

After agreement is reached concerning patient flows and priorities of off-service patients, the data of the pictorial summaries are used to construct the model for the hospital. It is not the purpose of this book to describe the detailed development of the model, but a brief explanation may be helpful. The following are the usual steps:

    a. A vector diagram of each unit is constructed that shows:

    1) Patient flows between units, patient flows entering units from outside the hospital representing hospital admissions and patient flows leaving the units representing hospital discharges. Patient flows for hospital admissions are determined for each unit for each type of

admission (emergency, urgent, and scheduled). Each patient flow vector entering a unit represents a segment of patient stay; i.e., a possible portion of a patient's entire hospital length of stay.

2) For all vectors, patient flow rates are determined from the data.

3) For all vectors implying admission or transfer to a unit the mean length of stay is determined from the data. Based on the product of the average LOS and average daily patient flow rate, each vector is assigned an average daily census (ADC).

4) From the vector diagram, the information required to properly size each unit is determined. This includes overall unit ADC, LOS, percent emergency, and percent scheduled.

5) From the vectors leaving units, a probability is computed to determine the next destination of the patients upon completing their current unit segment of stay.

b. Based on the number of units in the vector diagrams, a simulation model is created and initialized with each unit's bed capacities.

c. With day of the week specificity, the daily arrival rates for each unit's hospital admissions are determined and entered into the simulation model according to their type of admission. For emergencies, the arrival rates are also based on time of day of occurence.

d. With day of the week specificity, length of stay distributions are constructed from the data for every vector in the vector diagram and entered into the simulation model.

e. From the vector diagrams the next destination probability functions are entered into the simulation model.

f. The policies governing the priorities for off-service patients are entered into the simulation model.

g. For those vectors where Poisson arrival distributions are used (primarily emergent admissions), the weekly arrival rates are checked and adjusted via simulation

to match those in the vector diagaram. This process
is necessitated due to the use of random number
generators but does not consume much time because the
process has been automated.

   4.   Initial Model Validation

   Once the model is developed, initial results are obtained
from the simulator and checked against the data of the vector
diagram. The first results are used to determine the validity of
the model construction. The hypothesis is that if the model is
carefully and correctly built, the ADCs of the various units and
especially of the hospital as a whole will be the same as the ADC
computed for the vector diagrams. If they are within 1/2 patient
day, then we have assurances that the simulator can be used to
replicate the actual situation.

C.   Preliminary Decision Rules and Refinement of Systems
     Objectives

   Once the simulator is operational, preliminary decision
rules reflecting day-to-day operations under the ASCS can be
developed. The direction of this process, as specified at the
start of the project, is usually sufficient to guide initial
simulation efforts. With the creation of the vector diagram,
however, the validity of the initial project objectives is either
substantiated or challenged. Whichever the case, refinement of
system objectives involving hospital policies is often desirable.
Typical refinements are:

   1. Allocation of Excess Capacity

   In every implementation of the ASCS system, excess
capacities have been predicted to be available. Thus policies
are necessary to decide on how best to utilize these new excess
capacities. The hospital may want to do more surgery or provide
for the admission of more urgent patients or establish an
elective medical stream. There are, however, several factors
that should be taken into account when considering the best
policies to adopt. These are:

      a. That all of the clinical services, if possible,
         should get some benefit from the implementation of
         the system. For example, surgery may get reduced
         cancellations as well as an increase in scheduled
         admissions if the demand exists. Medicine may get an
         urgent call-in system so that they won't have to
         declare patients emergent to get them admitted.
         ICU/CCU may get priority in transferring their
         patients to acute units. For teaching hospitals,
         another objective might be to minimize the number of
         patients off-service for each specialty service.

b. For those services claiming to have additional demand
   to utilize the excess capacity, there should be some
   evidence that their increased capacity needs are
   real. There is a tendency for clinical services to
   claim potential future needs for additional capacity
   which do not always materialize. The ASCS system can
   handle some overstatement, but the overstatement will
   hasten the need to resimulate at an earlier future
   date than otherwise would be necessary if the demand
   does not materialize.

c. As a result of the discussions concerning a. & b.
   above, the need to resize various units and sub-units
   may become evident (see Chapter V). Though the
   resizing may not have an effect on overall system
   performance, it can have an effect on individual unit
   performance which is reflected in the simulation
   output statistics.

2. Setting the Elective Schedules

Frequently, the variation (based on the data collection) in
elective scheduled rates for each day of the week is high. One of
the ways the ASCS obtains higher occupancies is by establishing
set schedules for the admission of elective surgical patients.
In so doing, as many as or more elective surgeries can be
performed than in the past. In order to set these initial
surgical schedules and then to present and explain them to the
Executive Surgical Committee, operating room posting personnel
and hospital administration, analysis of the patient flow data is
helpful.

For example, Figure VI-3 is typical output from the initial
data analysis.

SUN	MON	TUE	WED	THU	FRI	SAT	TOTAL
18.7	16.6	15.2	15.7	14.4	0.7	0.3	81.6

Figure VI-3.   The Average Daily Admission Rate of Elective
                 Surgical Patients

Figure VI-4 might be an initial schedule. Please note that
the total elective patients scheduled is slightly higher (82 vs.
81.6) than the weekly average of the data base. Also, please
remember that the use of a schedule, like Figure VI-4, will
reduce the variance in number of admissions per day to very
nearly zero, while at the same time enabling slightly more
admissions than in the past.

```
SUN   MON   TUE   WED    THU    FRI   SAT   TOTAL
19    17    15    16     15      0     0     82
```

Figure VI-4 -- An Initial Schedule for Elective Surgical Cases

3. Analysis of Emergency Admissions

In order to determine the emergency admission rates to be used for each clinical unit, the average admission rates by day of the week are separated not only by clinical unit but also by type of emergent admission (direct and through the emergency room). These summaries are then used in the model development. Generally, these data are not presented to groups within the hospital because no decision is necessary. However, policy decisions do need to be made concerning the number of times per month that there will not be a bed available for emergent patients. Also, discussions concerning the ability to place patients in ICC/CCU overnight and/or to keep them in the emergency holding area of the emergency rooms or elsewhere in the hospital are necessary.

D. Simulator Ouput Using Initial Decision Rules

After deciding on the initial decision rules, a number of simulator runs are made to accomplish the objectives. Their results frequently lead to a series of "what if" questions concerning many different aspects of the operation of the hospital under the ASCS system. There seems to be no set pattern to these questions, but the following are a sample:

1. How much can we increase maximum average occupancy if we increase surgical cancellations to 3% from our initial specifications of 1%?

2. What will happen to occupancy if emergent patients can be admitted to ICU/CCU when beds are available?

3. If we resize the hospital units to be more consistent with the ADC of each unit, how much can we reduce the number of patients that are off-service?

4. What will happen to maximum average occupancy if we permit GYN Patients on the OB unit?

5. What will happen to maximum average occupancy if we change the age classification of pediatric patients from 14 to 19?

6. What would happen if we increase the size of the emergency holding area?

7. How many additional urgent patients can be admitted with our increased occupancy?

8. How many additional elective surgical patients can be admitted with the predicted increased occupancy?

9. How much higher could our occupancy be if some of our direct emergencies were converted to urgent admissions?

10. At what point does increasing our number of scheduled admissions seriously lower our potential maximum average occupancy?

Frequently the questions above again lead to extended discussions, but this time between the admissions personnel, administration, and physicians. After all of the issues are settled, the simulator is run to produce the final results. Usually at this point 200-week instead of 100-week runs of the simulation model are made with several random number seeds in order to make sure that the results are not random number seed dependent.

E.   Development of the Decision Tables

After the admissions decision numbers are developed, discussions are conducted in order to resolve the means and resources to monitor the ASCS system performance and the capability of personnel in terms of computer assistance and clerical staff to do so.
The decision tables are then developed (samples of these are in Chapter III). These tables are carefully reviewed with the admissions personnel in order to make sure of their clarity. Questions of clarity usually center around the definitions of words that are used. For example, in some hospitals, scheduled electives are called "guarantees" and emergent admissions are called "crises" or "necessary admissions." If these kinds of clarity problems exist, the decision rules are changed to use the vocabulary of the particular institution.

F.   Date of Implementation

An implementation date is chosen. Because elective surgeries are scheduled several weeks in advance, a date prior to the implementation date is decided upon after which O.R. posting personnel will be told to use the decision rules.

G.   Events Following Implementation

Weekly meetings are held following implementation to discuss any problems and answer questions raised by hospital personnel. The monitoring control charts are reviewed and discussed. Average occupancies are monitored to determine if the predicted results are being achieved. If not, investigations are conducted to determine the causes.

Any efforts required to assure the success of the implemented ASCS that have not yet been completed are pursued. These include:

1. Refinement of the historical data collection process so that resimulation efforts and costs for future years will be kept to a minimum.

2. Education of the hospital's management engineer or computer personnel in the use of the simulator and the hospital's model.

3. The training of the admissions personnel concerning how to modify the decision rules for holiday periods (Chapter III).

CHAPTER VII

THE DATA COLLECTION PROCESS

A.   Introduction

Upon embarking on any new effort involving state of the art technology, new concepts and nomenclature need to be mastered in order to assure the success of the project.   From the authors' experience this has proven to be true many times over, particularly in terms of implementations of the Admission Scheduling and Control System (ASCS).   Since the basic principles behind the ASCS had their start in industry, their associated concepts and nomenclature have essentially remained unchanged. However, because these principles invoke computer technology and apply them to a hospital environment, the creation of some new terminology has been unavoidable.

The purpose of this chapter is twofold in nature.   The first intent is to present the concepts and nomenclature that will be needed at the outset of ASCS implementation efforts.   This information is relevant for all members of the implementation team which normally includes at least one person from administration, management engineering, and data processing, as well as the chief admissions officer.   Following the presentation of the ASCS concepts and nomenclature, the data items to be collected are discussed in detail.

B.   The Model Construction Process

Once the decision is made to simulate a hospital's admission process, efforts are initiated to determine the appropriate model to be constructed for simulation.   Depending on the objectives, some times two or three variations (scenarios) of a model will be built and simulated.   These scenarios are generated for purposes of comparison and to determine an appropriate course of action to be taken.   In general these scenarios are very similar at the macro level but can differ substantially at the micro level.

The two basic premises of the simulation process are that the ASCS will be used as the admissions system and that the hospital's current patient mix and corresponding length of stays will be used in the simulation model.   In light of this, the intent of the simulation is to describe the hospital's potential given that the ASCS is implemented and then determine the appropriate ASCS parameters for implementation.

The process of creating a model involves two interrelated and dependent activities: 1) creating a model definition and 2) collecting the necessary data.   Neither activity can be pursued very far without information concerning the other.   To collect the data, information from the model definition is needed to determine what data to collect.   To set up the model definiton, knowledge of the hospital's operations, policies, objectives, layout, etc. are needed as well as an idea of what data are presently available for collection.   Often, the processing of the collected data reveals deficiencies in the model definition which in turn necessitates modification of the model definition and/or further manipulation of the collected data. It is also possible that additional data may need to be collected if the original data collection is determined to be incomplete.

C.   The Model Definition

A model definition is a structured set of rules that describe the logical collections of hospital beds and their associated patient flows into, between, and out of each of these collections of beds. In its early stages it begins without quantitative measures. It later becomes a simulation model when it is augmented by quantitative measures derived from the collected data and supplemented by policy directives to handle situations of insufficient bed availability.

Henceforth these "collections of beds" will be called units. To illustrate the flexibility of this unit concept the following groupings of beds could each be considered units: 1) a medical service, 2) an ICU, 3) a surgical specialty such as Plastic Surgery, 4) all surgical specialties comprising the service Surgery, 5) an emergency holding area, 6) selected floors of a hospital, 7) beds associated with selected nursing stations and 8) an entire hospital.

D.   The Block Diagram

In order to better conceptualize a particular model definition, an engineer draws a block diagram (see Figure VII-1) consisting of a number of boxes and arrows. Each box represents a unit and is labeled to indicate which beds and how many it represents. The arrows represent patient flows (or streams). The arrows with tails not attached to any unit represent patient arrival (admission) streams to the units from outside the hospital. Arrows with heads not pointing to any unit represent patient discharge streams associated with the units from which they originate. Arrows with both their heads and tails connected to units represent patient transfer streams between two units with the patient flow in the direction that the head indicates. Therefore there are three types of patient flow streams: 1) Admission, 2) Transfer, and 3) Discharge. These patient flow streams are also referred to as patient flow vectors or simply vectors. Excepting discharge vectors, each vector is associated with a segment of patient stay.

E.   The Patient Segment

Each patient's total hospital length of stay consists of one or more patient stay segments. The first of these segments is called the admission segment and all segments that follow are called transfer segments. By definition, a patient stay segment is associated with one and only one unit and continues until there is a change in this unit of association. The last of a patient's segments terminates upon discharge. The length of a

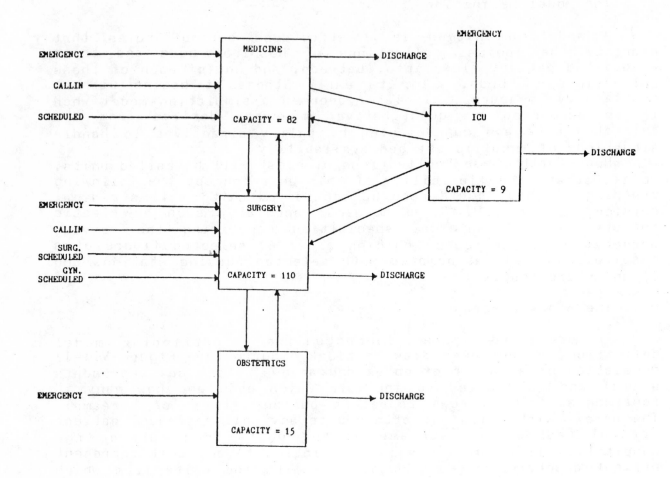

Figure VII-1 Block Diagram Illustrating Patient Flows
(Without Quantitative Measures)

segment is the amount of time that elapses between the start of the segment and the start of the next (or time of discharge if the segment in question is the last in the patient's hospital stay).

In Figure VII-2 some quantitative information has been added to the block diagram. For ASCS purposes, there are three types of admission streams (called admission types) possible for a unit from outside the hospital: 1) Emergency, 2) Call-in, and 3) Scheduled. These three admission types will be explained in more detail later. Note that it is possible to have more than one stream of each admission type into a unit.

The quantitative measures associated with the patient flow streams are as follows:

1. Average Arrival Rate on both a daily (ARR) and weekly (WKARR) basis.

2. Average Discharge Rate on both a daily (DIS) and weekly (WKDIS) basis.

3. Average Segment Length of Stay (LOS).

4. Average Daily Census (ADC). This statistic is calculated for a patient flow vector by: ADC = ARR X LOS. It indicates the number of beds on the unit that will be occupied on the average by the patients taking this method of admission to the unit for this segment of stay.

The block diagram appearing in Figure VII-3 is the result of programs using the collected data as input. Since an ASCS simulation model can have as many as 16 units and any number of admission and transfer vectors, the use of computer-generated block diagrams results in a significant savings of effort for the engineer, reduces the potential for errors, and also efficiently produces additional unit summary information. The following is a list of the conventions used in the production of the computer-generated block diagrams appearing in Figure VII-3.

1. Each unit in the block diagram is assigned a unit number which appears in the upper-right corner of the unit boxes.

2. All admission vectors appear on the left-hand side of the unit boxes.

3. All transfer vectors appear on the right-hand side of the unit boxes.

4. In lieu of having the tails of transfer vectors connected to their units of patient origination, labels are added to the tails to indicate unit origin.

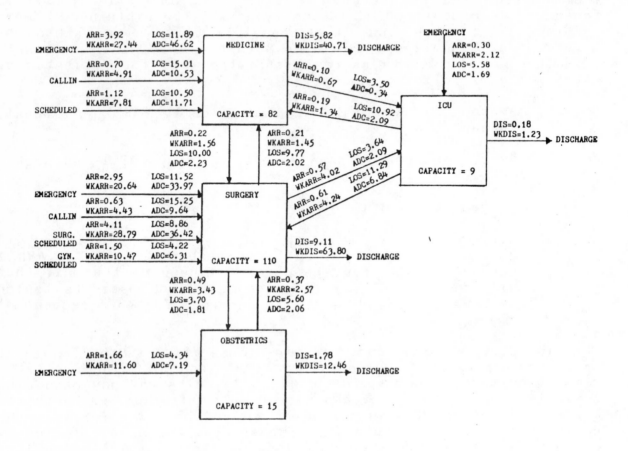

Figure VII-2   Block Diagram with Quantitative Measures

INTENSIVE/CARDIAC CARE UNIT (ICU_CCU) — 1

Left admission table:

TYPE OF ADMISSION	ARRIVAL RATES		MEAN LOS	AVG. DAILY CENSUS
	DAILY	WEEKLY		
EMERGENCY	0.303	2.120	5.58	1.689

OVERALL BREAKDOWN BY SUB-UNIT

SUB-UNIT	ARRIVAL RATES		MEAN LOS	AVG. DAILY CENSUS
	DAILY	WEEKLY		
ICU	0.749	5.242	4.00	2.996
CCU	0.223	1.562	5.00	1.115
TOTAL	0.972	6.804	4.23	4.111

DISCHARGE & TRANSFER BREAKDOWN

DESTINATION	AVERAGE RATES		% OF TOTAL
	DAILY	WEEKLY	
SURG	0.605	4.238	62.30
MED	0.191	1.338	19.67
DISCHARGE	0.175	1.227	18.03

CAP NOW = 9 | SIZED CAP =

Right transfer table:

ARRIVAL RATES		MEAN LOS	AVG. DAILY CENSUS	TRANSFERS FROM
DAILY	WEEKLY			
0.096	0.669	3.50	0.335	MED
0.574	4.015	3.64	2.087	SURG

MEDICINE UNIT (MED) — 2

Left admission table:

TYPE OF ADMISSION	ARRIVAL RATES		MEAN LOS	AVG. DAILY CENSUS
	DAILY	WEEKLY		
EMERGENCY	3.920	27.439	11.89	46.616
CALL-IN	0.701	4.908	15.01	10.525
SCHEDULED	1.115	7.807	10.50	11.711

OVERALL BREAKDOWN BY SUB-UNIT

SUB-UNIT	ARRIVAL RATES		MEAN LOS	AVG. DAILY CENSUS
	DAILY	WEEKLY		
MED1	1.386	9.704	15.02	20.826
MED2	0.207	1.450	9.93	2.056
MED3	4.079	28.554	10.82	44.153
MED4	0.462	3.235	12.82	5.927
TOTAL	6.135	42.942	11.89	72.962

DISCHARGE & TRANSFER BREAKDOWN

DESTINATION	AVERAGE RATES		% OF TOTAL
	DAILY	WEEKLY	
DISCHARGE	5.816	40.711	94.80
SURG	0.223	1.562	3.64
ICU_CCU	0.096	0.669	1.56

CAP NOW = 82 | SIZED CAP =

Right transfer table:

ARRIVAL RATES		MEAN LOS	AVG. DAILY CENSUS	TRANSFERS FROM
DAILY	WEEKLY			
0.191	1.338	10.92	2.087	ICU_CCU
0.207	1.450	9.77	2.024	SURG

Figure VII-3 Computer Generated Block Diagram

SURGERY UNIT
(SURG) | 3 |

OVERALL BREAKDOWN BY SUB-UNIT

SUB-UNIT	ARRIVAL RATES DAILY	WEEKLY	MEAN LOS	AVG. DAILY CENSUS
SURG1	2.103	14.723	7.64	16.062
SURG2	1.191	8.335	8.74	10.404
SURG3	0.749	5.242	6.45	4.828
SURG4	0.574	4.015	6.08	3.490
SURG5	0.685	4.796	13.93	9.544
SURG6	0.829	5.800	5.06	4.191
SURG7	2.071	14.500	14.28	29.573
SURG8	2.183	15.280	8.88	19.376
TOTAL	10.384	72.691	9.39	97.468

TYPE OF ADMISSION	ARRIVAL RATES DAILY	WEEKLY	MEAN LOS	AVG. DAILY CENSUS
EMERGENCY	2.948	20.635	11.52	33.971
CALL-IN	0.632	4.425	15.24	9.639
SURG_SCHED	4.113	28.791	8.86	36.423
GYN_SCHED	1.496	10.470	4.22	6.312

ARRIVAL RATES DAILY	WEEKLY	MEAN LOS	AVG. DAILY CENSUS	TRANSFERS FROM
0.605	4.238	11.29	6.836	ICU_CCU
0.223	1.562	10.00	2.231	MED
0.367	2.570	5.60	2.056	OBS

DISCHARGE & TRANSFER BREAKDOWN

DESTINATION	AVERAGE RATES DAILY	WEEKLY	% OF TOTAL
DISCHARGE	9.114	63.800	87.77
ICU_CCU	0.574	4.015	5.52
OBS	0.489	3.426	4.71
MED	0.207	1.450	1.99

| CAP NOW = 110 | SIZED CAP =

OBSTETRICS
(OBS) | 4 |

OVERALL BREAKDOWN BY SUB-UNIT

SUB-UNIT	ARRIVAL RATES DAILY	WEEKLY	MEAN LOS	AVG. DAILY CENSUS
OBS1	0.860	6.023	5.87	5.051
OBS2	1.286	9.003	3.07	3.952
TOTAL	2.147	15.026	4.19	9.003

TYPE OF ADMISSION	ARRIVAL RATES DAILY	WEEKLY	MEAN LOS	AVG. DAILY CENSUS
EMERGENCY	1.657	11.600	4.34	7.192

ARRIVAL RATES DAILY	WEEKLY	MEAN LOS	AVG. DAILY CENSUS	TRANSFERS FROM
0.489	3.426	3.70	1.811	SURG

DISCHARGE & TRANSFER BREAKDOWN

DESTINATION	AVERAGE RATES DAILY	WEEKLY	% OF TOTAL
DISCHARGE	1.779	12.456	82.90
SURG	0.367	2.570	17.10

| CAP NOW = 15 | SIZED CAP =

Figure VII-3 Computer Generated Block Diagram (Continued)

5. Since the tails of the transfer vectors are no longer physically connected to the unit of origin, a table called "DISCHARGE & TRANSFER BREAKDOWN" has been placed in the unit boxes to convey information about the next possible destinations for patients completing their present segments. This table is ordered by frequency of occurrence and reflects the same rates appearing in the corresponding transfer vectors.

6. The discharge vectors have been dropped entirely from the block diagram, but their information is retained in the "DISCHARGE & TRANSFER BREAKDOWN" tables.

7. Near the top of the unit boxes a table appears titled "OVERALL BREAKDOWN BY SUB-UNIT". Usually a data collection contains numberous sub-unit or service designations for its patients. Because of the small sizes of the many sub-units, economy of scale considerations and simulation restrictions, sub-units are often aggregated into single units on a many-to-one mapping basis. The vectors leading to a unit therefore represent the aggregates of the unit's sub-units' patient flows according to admission type or unit of origin of transfer. This table, however, displays the ARR, WKARRR, LOS, and ADC information for all admissions and transfers on a sub-unit basis. The bottom line of the table reflects the summary statistics for the entire unit which is the same whether calculated on a basis of all the unit's sub-units or vectors.

8. At the bottom of each unit box are spaces for two unit capacity values. The one on the left represents the unit's bed complement as it currently exists. The one on the right is reserved for the unit capacity indicated by the ASCS Bed Sizing Methodology (see Chapter V) based on the various unit quantitative measures also appearing in the unit box.

F. The Role Hospital Policies Play in a Model Definition

In Figure VII-4 another version of the block diagram is presented with symbols replacing the quantitative measures to indicate hospital policies. This version must be prepared prior to simulation, but has little bearing on the planning of the data collection. It cannot, however, be prepared until the basic model definition (without quantitative measures) is known.

The purpose of the policy block diagram is to answer the question "What happens to a patient trying to gain admission to a unit when no beds are available in the intended unit of admission?" To answer this question, the engineer establishes for each vector in the model a sequence of ALTERNATE ACTIONS to occur given that no beds are available in the intended unit of admission or transfer. Each alternate action is indicated by a diagonal arrow, a letter indicating the type of alternate action,

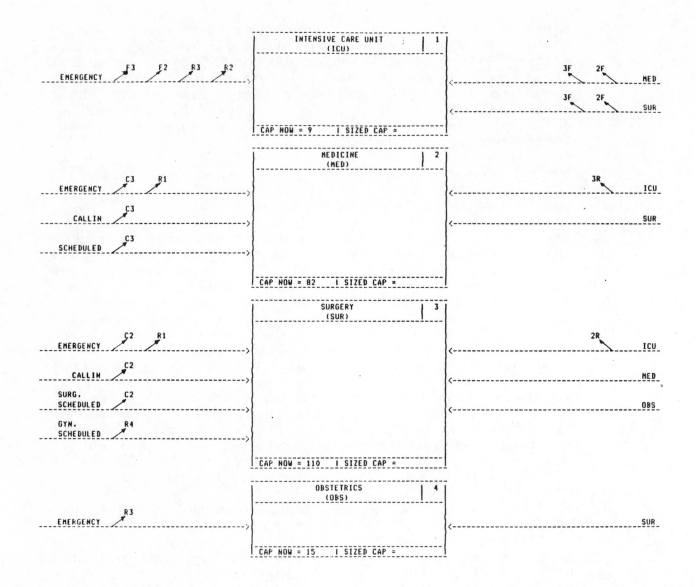

Figure VII-4 Block Diagram Indicating Policies of Handling
Insufficient Bed Availability Situations

and a unit's number against which the alterate action will be
processed. When necessary, these alternate actions are processed
in the order in which they appear when traversing the vector from
the tail to the head. Attempts to process each alternate action
in order continue until one is successfully executed or all have
failed. The three types of alternate actions are defined as
follows:

1. FORCE (F) -- This alternate action action attempts to
    find a patient (called the candidate) in the intended
    unit of admission who can be safely transferred (forced)
    to the unit indicated by the FORCE alternate action. If
    such a candidate is found and there is an available bed
    in the unit indicated by the alternate action, then a
    bed in the intended unit becomes available for the
    patient causing this FORCE and the alterate action is
    successful.

2. CO-UNIT REASSIGNMENT (C) -- This alternate action
    directs the patient to seek an available bed in the unit
    indicated by the alternate action (which is called the
    co-unit). If successful, the patient will remain
    associated with its intended unit but will reside in the
    co-unit for the duration of its segment's stay. An
    example of this co-unit reassignment is the assignment
    of a surgical patient to a medical bed for the first
    segment of the patient's hospital stay.

3. REDIRECTION (R) -- This alternate action directs the
    patient to seek an available bed in the unit indicated
    by the alternate action on a temporary basis. As soon
    as a bed becomes available in the patient's intended
    unit or one of its co-units, the patient is transferred
    to the empty bed. To illustrate this maneuver, say
    there are no beds available in Medicine or Surgery when
    an incoming Medical emergency patient is admitted to the
    hospital. Temporarily, the patient is given an ICU bed.
    When a patient is discharged from Medicine or Surgery
    later in the day, an empty bed is created and the
    Medicine patient in ICU is then transferred to the
    vacated bed in acute care.

Suppose a patient is attempting to gain admission to a unit
but no beds are available in this the (intended) unit and all
alternate actions (if any exist) have failed. If the patient is
an emergency patient attempting to start its first segment of
stay, then the patient is TURNED AWAY. Similarly, if the
patient is a scheduled patient attempting to start its first
segment of stay, then its admission is CANCELLED and must be
rescheduled for a later date. For patients attempting to
transfer following the completion of a segment of stay, the

patients are DELAYED on their present unit of residence and must attempt the transfer again at a later time. Note, the patient could not be a call-in patient, because the ASCS does not permit patients to be called in when no beds are available.

G.   Block Diagram Accuracy

As far as the basic model definition without quantitative measures is concerned, it must suit the objectives for simulation as well as present what the hospital's administration and admissions office feel is a true representation of the hospital and its patient flows. When the quantitative measures have been computed, the completeness and accuracy of the basic model definition will be known.

By checking other sources of information such as hospital occupancy and admission reports, verification is sought for the majority of the model's quantitative measures. This verification process begins at the macroscopic level and works down to the microscopic level. The first measure to be checked is the model's overall occupancy and average daily census which should differ by no more than one percent from the information supplied in the reports.   Next, the occupancies of the individual units are checked and then the individual patient flows if possible. Greater variation is permitted at this level because different assumptions may have been made in the methodologies used to compile the data collection and the hospital reports. However, gross differences must be investigated and corrected.   In a similar manner, the admission rates are also verified wherever possible.

As long as the quantitative measures are determined to be reasonably sound, simulations of the model and its scenarios will produce fairly accurate descriptions of the effects that the ASCS has on the hospital's admissions process.   Historically, the simulated model slightly understates (up to one percent) the benefits of ASCS implementations due to the fact that more options are available to the admissions officer than are feasible to simulate.

Since the policy block diagram is produced in concert with a hospital's admissions officer and administration representative, the diagram should be quite accurate.   It is the responsibility of the engineer to make sure that the information and its use are understood by each person involved in the design of the policy block diagram.

H.   The Effects of a Hospital's Non-ASCS Admission Types on the Project

The fact that a hospital does not maintain the same types of admission as used by the ASCS should not pose a problem for implementation since most hospitals' admission types are simple variations or subsets of the ASCS admission types.   To demonstrate this, the three ASCS admission types are discussed below in this light:

1. EMERGENCY -- A patient is classified as an emergency
    only if there is a bonafide need for immediate hospital
    admission. To date, three different hospital admission
    types have fallen into this category: 1) Emergency, 2)
    Direct Admits also called Crisis (usually patients sent
    directly to the hospital from a doctor's office) and 3)
    Through Emergency Room. In each case, the admissions
    office has no way either to control or know in advance
    how many of these patients will seek admission on any
    given day.

2. CALL-IN -- This type of admission is given to those
    patients who not only do not need an immediate admission
    upon request, but also permit the hospital to call them
    in for admission at the hospital's convenience (subject
    to the urgency of the patient's condition). To date,
    Urgent   and   Elective   (where   elective   implies
    non-scheduled) have been the labels on the hospitals'
    admission types that fall into the CALL-IN category.

3. SCHEDULED -- This admission type is given to those
    patients who have been given a fixed date in the future
    for admission by the hospital and then admitted on that
    date. This category of patients has received the
    following labels by various hospitals: 1) Scheduled, 2)
    Planned, 3) Guaranteed, and 4) Elective (where elective
    implies non-call-in).

I. Other Data Collections That Will Be Required for ASCS
    Implementation

    For the construction of the model, the following is a list
of other data to be collected:

1. Time of day that each patient stay segment begins. This
    information is a part of the quantitative measures data
    collection.

2. Time of day that each patient is discharged from the
    hospital.   This information is a part of the
    quantitative measures data collection.

3. A determination of the average number of beds
    out-of-service daily for each unit of the model due to
    reasons of isolation-patients in a double room, bed
    maintenance, repair, etc. Beds out-of-service for any
    lengthy duration of time due to shutdown of a nursing
    station, insufficient staffing, or for other
    administrative reasons should be reflected in the units'
    capacities and not in the average numbers of beds
    out-of-service.

4. A survey of the average number and types of surgical
operations performed on each day of the week. This
information will be required just prior to simulation so
that schedules for admission to surgical units can be
coordinated with the activities of the operating rooms.

If there is a substantial time lag between the quantitative
measures data collection and the installation of the ASCS, a
second set of data may be required to adjust for any arrival
rates that change.

Following the installation of the ASCS, it will be necessary
to collect various data items to monitor the system. Should
these data indicate that a significant change has occurred in
either the vector arrival rates and/or patient mix, then once
again it will be necessary to resimulate. Resimulation may or
may not require additional data collection. However,
resimulation is suggested every two or three years based on new
data collections. The implications of these resimulation and
potential new data collections are that upon project initiation,
plans should be made to start an ongoing data collection.

For the purposes of simulation, only three months of
quantitative measures data are required, though six or more
months of data are desirable. Prior to implementation of the
ASCS, a total of six months (preferably nine) of the quantitative
measures data is necessary to set up various prediction tools for
the ASCS decision process.

J.   Specifications for the Quantitative Measures Data Collection

      1. The ASCS Service

      The essence of the quantitative measures data collection is
to procure an accurate and recent historical collection of data
in which each patient's hospital stay is tracked in terms of the
patient's "need for an ASCS service." The ASCS service is
defined as that portion of the hospital's bed complement in which
the patient SHOULD BE residing in order to most efficiently and
effectively receive the proper care. All ASCS service categories
are mutually exclusive. The data collection must indicate for
each patient the dates and times of day that a particular need
for an ASCS service begins and ends. Each patient hospital stay
will therefore consist of one or more segments of stay. The
first segment of stay begins at admission and the last ends with
discharge. If, at any point in a patient's hospital stay, the
patient's need for an ASCS service changes, then one segment of
stay ends and a new one begins. Segments of stay following the
initial segment beginning at admission are called "transfer
segments."

      Upon initiation of the request for the data collection, it
is unusual to find a hospital's data base containing a single
field in which the ASCS service definition is completely
satisfied. The field traditionally called "hospital service"
usually fails the definition when used by itself because it does

not identify intensive care or coronary care units as services. Similarly, when used alone, the field called "bed service" or "nursing station," indicating general location of a patient's bed, yields an invalid result if a patient is located off-service. Finally, some hospitals need to have the ASCS service field identify specific teams of resident physicians responsible for patients and this identification is not currently a part of their computer's hospital service field. As a result, a field indicating the attending physician must also be used in the determination of the ASCS services.

Earlier in this chapter, the patient segment was defined in terms of the units that make up the block diagram. That definition is still valid but it portrays the macroscopic view of the model. In the discussion of the block diagram produced by computer processing of the data collection, the term "sub-unit" was introduced. For most applications, there is a one-to-one correspondence between the ASCS services and the sub-units in the block diagrams. When this is not the case, then there is a many-to-one mapping of ASCS services into sub-units.

One might conclude that the level of detail required for the ASCS service is considerable. The problem is that if the presently collected data do not provide a sufficient understanding of the patient flows, then a new data collection will be necessary in order for the simulator to accurately reflect what is happening. The data requirements for teaching hospitals are more demanding than those of the community hospitals because they are more dynamic in their policies and have a tendency to reorganize their services as well as introduce new clinical specialties. This often results in a need to add new schedule streams (and sometimes units) to their simulation model. This is a fairly routine matter, assuming that the level of detail currently exists in the data to identify the new stream or unit components. However, if the detail is not sufficient, new data must be collected.

As an example, Figure VII-5 illustrates the ASCS services within Hospital "XYZ" that were proposed for its data collection.

2. Data Collection Methodologies

a. The Ideal Method of Transmission and Data Structure

The best method to capture the data collection is to obtain it directly from the hospital's own computer data base, assuming that it exists and is complete as far as the desired fields are concerned. In so doing, errors will be kept to a minimum and so will the time and money associated with the data collection. Figure VII-6 illustrates the ideal data structure for the data capture and transmission. This is a PL/I based data structure that makes use of the "REFER" option, thus permitting the inclusion of a variable number of transfer data segments (TRAN_SEGS) with every patient stay record. For the majority of patient records, there should be no transfer segments and the "#_OF_TRANS_SEG" field would contain a zero. When a patient record does require the transfer segment portion of the data

ITEM #	ABBREVIATION	DESCRIPTION
1	MEDA	MEDICINE A
2	MEDB	MEDICINE B
3	DER	DERMATOLOGY
4	RAD	RADIATION THERAPY
5	SURG	SURGERY (GENERAL)
6	CRCT	COLON-RECTAL (PROCTOLOGY)
7	ENT	EAR, NOSE, AND THROAT
8	GYN	GYNECOLOGY
9	HAND	HAND SURGERY
10	OPT	OPHTHALMOLOGY
11	ORT	ORTHOPEDICS
12	PLAS	PLASTIC SURGERY
13	THOR	THORACIC SURGERY
14	URO	UROLOGY
15	VAS	VASCULAR SURGERY
16	ONCA	ONCOLOGY A
17	ONCB	ONCOLOGY B
18	PALL	PALLIATIVE
19	NEU	NEUROLOGY
20	NSU	NEURO-SURGERY
21	FPR	FAMILY PRACTICE
22	3ICU	INTENSIVE CARE UNIT ON 3WT (THOR/CADIO POST OP)
23	ONCS	SPECIAL CARE UNIT ON 4WT FOR ONCOLOGY
24	5ICU	INTENSIVE CARE UNIT ON 5WT (VAS & GEN SURG ICU)
25	6ICU	CORONARY CARE UNIT ON 6WT
26	8ICU	INTENSIVE CARE UNIT ON 8WT (NEU/NSU ICU)
27	9ICU	INTENSIVE CARE UNIT ON 9WT (MEDICINE ICU)
28	XICU	INTENSIVE CARE UNIT ON 10WT (MED/SURG ICU)
29	PSY	PSYCHIATRY
30	ALCO	ALCOHOL TREATMENT

Figure VII-5   Breakdown of The ASCS Service Catagories
for Hospital "XYZ" Data Collection

record, it more than likely will contain only one or two transfer segments. On rare occasions, a patient will require as many as seven or eight transfer segments.

```
DCL    1 ASCS_DATA_STRUCTURE    BASED(ASCS_PTR),
         2 PATIENT_ID              CHAR(8),
         2 ADMIT_DATE              CHAR(6),
         2 ADMIT_TIME              CHAR(4),
         2 ADM_ASCS_SERVICE        CHAR(4),
         2 TYPE_OF_ADM             CHAR(1),
         2 PATIENT_AGE             CHAR(3),
         2 PATIENT_SEX             CHAR(1),
         2 ADMIT_PHYS              CHAR(4),
         2 ATTEND_PHYS             CHAR(4),
         2 PRIMARY_DIAG            CHAR(5),
         2 SUR_NONSUR_PROC         CHAR(4),
         2 DISCHARGE_DATE          CHAR(6),
         2 DISCHARGE_TIME          CHAR(4),
         2 #_OF_TRANS_SEG          BINARY FIXED(15,0),
         2 TRAN_SEGS(#TOALL REFER(3_OF_TRANS_SEG)),
              3 TRANSFER_DATE         CHAR(6),
              3 TRANSFER_TIME         CHAR(4),
              3 TRANS_ASCS_SERVICE    CHAR(4);
```

Figure VII-6   An Ideal Data Structure

The following is a key to each of the data fields appearing in the data structure in Figure VII-6:

PATIENT_ID -- This field contains a unique number associated with the patient. In some hospitals this number is patient-specific and is the same each time the patient is admitted to the hospital. In other hospitals, this number is unique for every hospital stay. It makes no difference which system is used or even if the number is scrambled for security purposes, as long as the PATIENT_ID and admission date together indicate a particular patient hospital stay and that the original medical records of corresponding patients' stays can be identified if necessary. With this ability to uniquely identify each patient stay, two benefits are achieved: 1) any data problems that arise are more easily traceable and resolved and 2) if additional data are collected for other systems work, then they can be linked with the historical data collection (assuming it uses the same patient stay identification).

ADMIT_DATE -- This field contains the date the patient was admitted to the hospital and has the format MMDDYY where: "MM" is the month, "DD" is the day of the month and "YY" is the year.

ADMIT_TIME -- This field contains the time of day that the patient was admitted to the hospital and has a format of HHMM where "HHMM" is the time of day in military time.

ADM_ASCS_SERVICE -- This field contains the code for the ASCS service the patient needs upon admission to the hospital. This ASCS service is associated with the admission segment of stay.

TYPE_OF_ADM -- this field contains the type of admission for the patient admission as recorded by the admissions department. For example, let: 1=Emergency, 2=Urgent, 3=Elective, 4=Direct.

PATIENT_AGE -- This field contains the patient's age in years at the time of admission.

PATIENT_SEX -- This optional field contains an indication of the patient's sex; i.e., "1" or "M" for male and "2" or "F" for female.

ADMIT_PHYS -- This optional field contains the physician code used by the hospital to indicate the patient's admitting physician.

ATTEND_PHYS -- This optional field contains the physician code used by the hospital to indicate the patient's primary attending physician during the course of the patient's hospital stay.

PRIMARY_DIAG -- This optional field contains the primary ICD-9-CM code for the diagnosis best describing need for hospital stay. Codes should be entered such that the implied decimal point is between the third and forth position from the left.

SUR_NONSUR_PROC -- This optional field contains the ICD-9-CM code for the principal surgical or nonsurgical procedure performed on the patient during the hospital stay. If none, then leave blank. Codes should be entered such that the implied decimal point is between the second and third position.

DISCHARGE_DATE -- This field contains the date the patient was discharged from the hospital and has the format MMDDYY where: "MM" is the month, "DD" is the day of the month and "YY" is the year.

DISCHARGE_TIME -- This field contains the time of day that the patient was discharged from the hospital and has a format of HHMM where "HHMM" is the time of day in military time.

#_OF_TRANS_SEG -- This field contains the number of transfer segments to follow that are associated with the admission/discharge portion of the patient stay record. The field has a length of two bytes and contains a binary number greater than or equal to zero.

TRANSFER_DATE -- This field will appear for each transfer segment and contains the date the transfer segment begins. The format for the field is MMDDYY where: "MM" is the month, "DD" is the day of the month and "YY" is the year.

TRANSFER_TIME -- This field will appear for each transfer segment and contains the time of day that the transfer segment begins. The format for the field is HHMM where "HHMM" is the time of day in military time.

TRANS_ASCS_SERVICE -- This field will appear for each transfer segment and contains the ASCS service code associated with the transfer segment.

It is not mandatory that the data structure presented in Figure VII-6 be followed verbatim since data as well as computing hardware and software vary from one hospital to another. It is essential, however, that each field in the data transmitted adheres to the definitions from above and that all fields not specified as optional be present.

b. Data Collections Using Abstracting Services

Many hospitals already participate in data abstraction arrangements in conjunction with outside computer service organizations. Depending on the complexity of the hospital and the data to be captured by the abstract forms, copies of the abstracted data (transmitted via computer magnetic tape) may satisfy a major portion of the ASCS data collection requirements. Unfortunately, there are a number of problems usually associated with this arrangemnt due to the fact that the data to be abstracted are dictated by the computer service organization and are intended as input for their "canned" programs. Some of the problems that this causes are:

1) Assumptions may be required in the processing of the data for ASCS purposes. This is particularly true for service and type-of-admission fields for which the abstract's definitions are frequently in conflict with those of the ASCS.

2) The abstracted data do not usually track patient stays in terms of patient stay segments as defined by the ASCS. As a result, a number of assumptions are required to determine patient flows between units. For a major teaching hospital, this can be a major obstacle.

3) Because the data abstraction process is often established primarily to satisfy legal requirements, many of the reports produced by the computer service organization are not carefully scrutinized. Errors escaping the normal computer editing procedures go undetected and are perpetuated month after month. Unlike the summary reports for which these data are abstracted, these errors can be misleading in the construction of an ASCS model.

4) Other sources of error include abstractors' misinterpretation of patient records which may be either complete at the time and/or misleading. Stray marks on the abstract forms as well as coding that is too light can cause the optical reading machinery to produce erroneous records that still pass edit checking.

In general, if the data collection is to be based on patient record abstracts, then additional data will be required to verify the validity of the data.

c. Data Collections by Brute Force

When other alternatives are not available, the data collection must be obtained by "brute force." This is the least desirable of the three alternatives because it is by far the most expensive and potentially the least accurate. Another fact to consider is that there will also be a need for an ongoing historical data collection following implementation.

The "brute force" method involves the design of a process where a number of data sources are to be merged in order to produce the individual patient records of the data collection. The data sources may include admission/discharge/transfer reports, ICU/CCU logs, emergency room logs, and ultimately the patient medical records.

The most efficient way to capture the data is to aggregate each individual patient record on a form which is then submitted for keypunching (for 80-column computer cards), key-to-disk transcription, or key-to-tape transcription. The advantage of key-to-disk and key-to-tape over keypunching is that there is essentially no restriction on the length of the data record. With computer cards, those patient records having transfer segments may require two or more cards. This has the drawback that multiple cards per patient record must each include patient stay identification (medical or patient record number and admission date) as well as a field indicating the intended sequential order of the cards within the patient record. Without such identification, erroneous duplications cannot be checked and a dropped card deck would probably result in a substantial amount of wasted effort.

In Figure VII-7, two 80-column card formats are presented as an example of a combination data collection and keypunching form. The first card contains the information pertaining to the

CARD #1:   PATIENT ADMISSION/DISCHARGE DATA AND PATIENT DEMOGRAPHICS

C A R D	PATIENT IDENTIFICATION NUMBER OR MEDICAL RECORD NUMBER	ADMISSION					T Y P A D	AGE	S E X	ADMIT SVC	ADMISSION LOCATION	DISCHARGE					PRIMARY DIAGNOSIS	PRINCIPAL SURGICAL PROCEDURE
		DATE			TIME							DATE			TIME			
1		MONTH	DAY	YEAR	HOUR	MIN.						MONTH	DAY	YEAR	HOUR	MIN.		

1 2 3 4 5 6 7 8 9 0   1 2 3 4 5 6 7 8 9 0   1 2 3 4 5 6 7 8 9 0   1 2 3 4 5 6 7 8 9 0   1 2 3 4 5 6 7 8 9 0
              1   2   3   4   5

                              FIRST TRANSFER SEGMENT DATA

ADMITTING PHYSICIAN	PRINCIPAL ATTENDING PHYSICIAN	TRANSFER					TRANS SVC	TRANSFER LOCATION	UNUSED
		DATE			TIME				
		MONTH	DAY	YEAR	HOUR	MIN.			

1 2 3 4 5 6 7 8 9 0   1 2 3 4 5 6 7 8 9 0   1 2 3 4 5 6 7 8 9 0
              6   7   8

CARD #2:   PATIENT TRANSFER SEGMENT DATA CONTINUED

C A R D	PATIENT IDENTIFICATION NUMBER OR MEDICAL RECORD NUMBER	ADMISSION DATE			2ND TRANSFER SEGMENT							3RD TRANSFER SEGMENT						
					TRANSFER					TRANS SVC	TRANSFER LOCATION	TRANSFER					TRANS SVC	TRANSFER LOCATION
					DATE			TIME				DATE			TIME			
		MONTH	DAY	YEAR	MONTH	DAY	YEAR	HOUR	MIN.			MONTH	DAY	YEAR	HOUR	MIN.		

1 2 3 4 5 6 7 8 9 0   1 2 3 4 5 6 7 8 9 0   1 2 3 4 5 6 7 8 9 0   1 2 3 4 5 6 7 8 9 0   1 2 3 4 5 6 7 8
              1   2   3   4

4TH TRANSFER SEGMENT							5TH TRANSFER SEGMENT						
TRANSFER					TRANS SVC	TRANSFER LOCATION	TRANSFER					TRANS SVC	TRANSFER LOCATION
DATE			TIME				DATE			TIME			
MONTH	DAY	YEAR	HOUR	MIN.			MONTH	DAY	YEAR	HOUR	MIN.		

9 0 1 2 3 4 5 6 7 8 9 0   1 2 3 4 5 6 7 8 9 0   1 2 3 4 5 6 7 8 9 0
            5   6   7   8

Figure VII-7 Examples of Double Card Data Format of Patient Flow Data

patient's overall hospital stay and a first transfer segment (if necessary). The second card format can be used for all subsequent patient transfer segments, though it is designed for second through fifth patient transfer segments. By placing a "3" in column #1, the card will imply segments 6,7,8 and/or 9. As a matter of definition, the abbreviation "TPAD" stands for type of admission, "ADMIT SVC" stands for patient service for the admission segment of stay, and "TRANS SVC" stands for patient service of the transfer segment.

Note, these card formats capture both patient service and patient location instead of "ASCS service" for each patient stay segment (patient location may be defined by nursing station, bed service, or room/bed number). With this approach it is necessary to define a new transfer segment every time the patient service or patient location changes. This strategy requires that the computer used to analyze the data also determine the ASCS service based on the combination of patient service, patient location, and possibly attending physician. This can be advantageous when it is unclear at the start of implementation what the hospital's ASCS services should be. Though this adds a degree of flexibility, it also increases the time requirements for analysis due to the increased level of complexity.

In addition to those disadvantages already presented for the "brute force" methodology, errors due to keypunching must be expected. For those that can be detected during analysis, correction should be attempted in lieu of discarding obviously erroneous data.

3. Data Transfer Medium Specifications

The best medium for data transfer is half inch, 9 track, 1600 or 6250 BPI magnetic computer tape using EBCDIC codes for the character fields. It is preferable that the tape be labeled using the IBM OS/VS labeling scheme; otherwise the tape should be unlabeled. A "VBS" tape format is preferable to a "U" tape format though either is acceptable.

Though 80-column computer cards are a possible data transfer medium, their unwieldiness leaves much to be desired. It is preferable that the card images be recorded on computer tape according to the specifications presented in the previous paragraph. Since computer cards are a fixed length medium, a fixed length and blocked (FB) tape format might be used in lieu of the "VBS" tape format.

4. Data Retention

Though it is possible to use data from as few as six months of discharges when processing for the ASCS, best results are obtained when the data include all discharges spanning a calendar year. As a result, it is advisable to retain the data collection for all discharges back to and including the last complete calendar year.

CHAPTER VIII

ASCS-II SIMULATOR: DOCUMENTATION FOR THE ENGINEER

A. Introduction

This chapter is designed to aid hospital management engineers and other technical personnel in the operation of the Admission Scheduling and Control System Simulator II (ASCS-II). It is not intended to cover all aspects of the simulator's functions and capabilities since that is the purpose of the manual, "Admission Scheduling and Control System Simulator II: Documentation for Developing ASCS Simulation Models" (1). Instead, it is designed to assist in simulator operation for hospital inpatient admissions system models already in use but in need of resimulation because of dynamic changes in the inpatient flows of the hospital.

Both the simulation process and the ability to make minor alterations to the simulation model are important aspects of ASCS maintenance and should be mastered by one or more members of the hospital's management engineering or computer departments, preferably the person(s) overseeing the technical aspects of the admissions operations. By having the hospital's own personnel develop in-house expertise, the following benefits can be realized:

1. Many of the "what if" type of questions concerning the implementation coming from administration, physicians, the admissions office, etc. can be answered from within the hospital.

2. Because the admissions process has periods of high and low demand, there will be pressure exerted by various members of the hospital community to "temporarily" alter the ASCS allowances to accommodate the immediate situation. Having performed the ASCS simulations, the in-house experts will be prepared to defend the ASCS allowances which in conjunction with the ASCS algorithms are specifically designed to handle the normal fluctuations in demand. At times, however, it is necessary to "temporarily" override the ASCS allowances, but to do so without an adequate understanding of the system dynamics can result in greater problems within a few days or weeks in terms of cancellations, turnaways, and lower overall occupancy.

3. Additions to and departures from the hospital's staff of physicians normally do not cause change in hospital policy; however, they can significantly affect admission

rates. With in-house expertise, resimulation can be performed without delay so that the ASCS decision numbers can be modified to reflect the changes in admission rates.

4. Having simulated the hospital's admission system, the in-house experts will be able to increase both the viability and value of the implemented ASCS:

    a. Monitoring tools built into the ASCS can be interpreted to determine the adequacy of the current allowances.

    b. Periodic training sessions for admissions office personnel can be performed promptly.

    c. By insuring that the ASCS is functioning smoothly, the viability of other systems dependent on a stable admissions function is increased. This includes such systems as pre-admission testing, housekeeping, operating room scheduling and nurse staffing.

B. Computing Equipment Requirements

The computing equipment needed to operate the ASCS-II is a computer terminal and either a modem or acoustic coupling device which permits the terminal to be connected to the phone lines. It is possible to use a CRT (television screen) type of terminal, though it is not advisable since hard copy output can facilitate the simulation process significantly. Terminals capable of 132-column output are preferable to those capable of displaying a maximum of 80 columns. With 80 columns a large portion of the descriptive text included in the simulation output will have to be significantly abbreviated, truncated, or permitted to wrap around from one line to the next.

C. The Michigan Terminal System

ASCS-II is currently implemented on the University of Michigan's Amdahl V/8 computer in Ann Arbor, Michigan. The operating system environment in which the simulator runs is called the Michigan Terminal System (MTS). MTS is operational on a 24 hour per day basis, seven days per week, with occasional early morning (6 A.M. to 7 A.M.) downtime for maintenance purposes. During the period of 8 A.M. to 5 P.M., MTS experiences its heaviest load which may result in slow program execution; however, the execution speed of the simulator during this time period is not intolerable.

D. Establishing a Connection with MTS

To gain access to MTS, the user must first be issued a computer communication identification (CCID) and a password for that CCID. Arrangements for obtaining the CCID and password can be made through the authors. Next, the method of establishing the connection with MTS must be chosen. For those users able to make local phone calls to Ann Arbor, two options exist: either a full-duplex connection or a half-duplex connection. The following sequence will establish the full-duplex connection for terminals that operate at either 30 characters per second (300 Baud) or 120 characters per second (1200 Baud):

1. Turn on terminal. If an acoustic coupler is being used, do not turn it on at this time.
2. Make sure that any off-line/on-line switch is in the on-line switch setting.
3. Turn the full/half duplex switch on the terminal to the "full" position.
4. Dial (313) 763-4800 for terminals operating at 30 characters per second (300 Baud) or dial (313) 763-6500 for terminals operating at 120 characters per second (1200 Baud).
5. For those using acoustic couplers, place the phone in the coupler when the high-pitched carrier tone is heard. For those using a modem connected to a phone with a switch-hook, dial the phone number above with the phone in voice mode and then, when the high-pitched carrier tone is heard, engage the data mode and leave the phone off the hook.
6. If a coupler is being used, turn it on now.
7. Wait until two noise characters appear and then depress the carriage return.
8. Now enter the "terminal type" followed by a carriage return. Terminal types such as LA36, LA120, TTY33, AJ830, GE300, etc. identify the type of terminal being used to the system. If you do not know the terminal type, then contact the authors or the University of Michigan Computing Center.
9. A message to the effect of "MTS Ann Arbor" plus a series of letters and numbers enclosed in parentheses will be printed. When the MTS mode prompting character "#" appears, proceed to sign on as directed below.

The following sequence will establish a half-duplex connection for terminals that operate at 30 characters per second (300 Baud).

1. Turn on terminal. If an acoustic coupler is being used, do not turn it on at this time.

2. Make sure that any off-line/on-line switch is in the on-line switch setting.

3. Turn the full/half duplex switch on the terminal to the "half" position.

4. Dial (313) 763-0300.

5. Place the phone in the coupler when the high pitched carrier tone is heard.

6. Turn on the coupler.

7. Type: "GO" followed by a carriage return.

8. Now enter the "terminal type" followed by a carriage return. Terminal types such as LA36, LA120, TTY33, AJ830, GE300, etc. identify the type of terminal being used to the system. If you do not know the terminal type, then contact the authors or the University of Michigan Computing Center.

9. A message to the effect of "MTS Ann Arbor" plus a series of letters and numbers enclosed in parentheses will be printed. When the MTS mode prompting character "#" appears, proceed to sign on as directed below.

For those users unable to make local calls to Ann Arbor, the above two methods will also work, though the phone call will have to be long distance. Because of noise problems in long distance calls, the full-duplex type of connection seems to be the better access method. As an attractive alternative to the expense of accessing MTS via long distance phone calls, it is possible to establish a connection with MTS through the Telenet-Merit Network by means of dialing a local GTE Telenet access phone number. If this is possible, then the user will have an additional charge for Telenet-Merit Network connect time of approximately ten dollars per hour automatically added to the computer charges in lieu of a long distance phone charge. To access MTS via the Telenet-Merit Network, the user is advised to obtain a copy of the "Merit Computer Network User's Memo No. 12" (2). This memo is not essential, but it does contain local Telenet phone numbers around the country, lists of Telenet IDs for terminals and other helpful information concerning the use of the Telenet-Merit Network connections not covered in this chapter. The following is a synopsis of the procedures necessary to access MTS via the Telenet-Merit Network:

1. Turn on terminal. If an acoustic coupler is being used, do not turn it on at this time.

2. Make sure that any off-line/on-line switch is in the on-line switch setting.

3. Turn the full/half duplex switch on the terminal to the "full" position.

4. Dial the local Telenet phone number. A list of local Telenet phone numbers for all areas of the United States appears in the "Merit Computer Network User's Memo No. 12" (2).

5. Place the phone in the coupler when the high-pitched carrier tone is heard.

6. Turn on the coupler.

7. Depress the carriage return twice.

8. Telenet will identify itself and inquire about the type of terminal being used. Type in the four-character Telenet ID for the terminal followed by a carriage return. The "Merit Computer Network User's Memo No. 12" (2) contains a listing of all acceptable Telenet IDs.

9. Telenet will prompt you with an at-sign "@". Type a "C" for "connect," skip a space, and type the address number "31362" of the Merit Network, followed by a carriage return.

10. Telenet will respond with a connection message.

11. You will then be prompted with "Which host?" to which "UM" followed by a carriage return will connect you with MTS.

12. A message to the effect of "MTS Ann Arbor" plus a series of letters and numbers enclosed in parentheses will be printed. When the MTS mode prompting character "#" appears, proceed to sign on as directed below.

E. Signing on MTS

With the appearance of the MTS prompting character "#" following the "MTS Ann Arbor (....)" message, the user has five minutes to "SIGNON" to MTS. This MTS command identifies the user to MTS and initiates the terminal session. It should be issued as follows:

    $SIGNON ccid

followed by a carriage return, where "ccid" is the user's signon ID (Computer Communications ID number).
    After the SIGNON command is entered, the user is prompted to enter the password that has been previously set for the user's ccid. This password is a security measure to insure that only the users authorized to use this ccid gain access to MTS via this ccid. The password is a string of up to twelve characters and/or numbers (no blanks). The prompting sequence for the user password is as follows:

    #ENTER USER PASSWORD
    ?

If the user has made a half-duplex connection to MTS, then the twelve characters following the "?" will be blanked out by a series of characters overprinting on themselves and the user's password will be hidden when entered. For other types of connections to MTS, the printing of the password will simply be suppressed when entered. Follow the password with a carriage return to send it to MTS. If the password is incorrect, then MTS will print:

        #PASSWORD INCORRECT. TRY AGAIN
        ?

MTS will give the user three chances to get the password right before dropping the connection.

After the correct password has been entered, MTS will again issue the MTS mode prompting character "#" at which point the user is signed onto MTS and can proceed with the terminal session.

For the rest of this chapter specific instructions concerning "carriage returns" will be omitted. It should be understood that a line of information or a command to be entered by the user is transmitted to the computer only when the carriage return key is depressed. Prior to transmission, a line of user input may be back-spaced and retyped or deleted and completely reentered. Hereafter, in references to command entries, user responses to prompting messages, and other forms of user input to the computer, it will be assumed that a carriage return always follows the line of input.

F. MTS -- a Few Selected Topics and Commands

In the course of running the ASCS-II, a small amount of interaction with MTS will be necessary if the user wants to minimize his/her efforts during the simulation process. Without such interaction, the user may face a significant amount of repetitive reinitialization when simulating a single model over a number of terminal sessions. It is unnecessary for the user to be well versed in the intricacies of MTS, but a grasp of a few concepts and commands dealing with the manipulation of files is important. This section will therefore present a brief overview of selected aspects of MTS (see MTS Volume #1 (3) for greater detail).

1. MTS Files

Associated with each ccid account is an allocation of money and permanent disk file storage space (or simply filespace). As long as there is money in the account, the user can continue to operate on the ccid. Similarly, as long as the user has not exceeded the allotted amount of filespace for the ccid, then more files may be constructed and existing files expanded. When the

allotted filespace is exceeded, either some of the permanent
files on the ccid must be destroyed or the filespace allotment
increased in order to permanently save additional information in
disk files.

In addition to the permanent filespace allotted to the ccid,
the user has an almost unlimited amount of temporary filespace at
his/her disposal during the course of a terminal session. The
information stored in temporary files, however, is lost upon
completing the terminal session.

Whether a file has a permanent or temporary status, a file
is either a "line file" or a "sequential file." ASCS-II makes
use of both types. Each ASCS-II simulation model that is stored
on disk has one part of the model stored in a line file and the
other part stored in a sequential file. All other files
associated with ASCS-II are line files. It is not important that
the user understand the nature of these two file types, only when
and where to use them.

All files have names. The names of permanent files consist
of one to twelve characters. The name may contain letters
(lowercase letters are automatically converted to uppercase),
digits, and special characters (excepting: ,;:()@+='"?& and
blank). Names for temporary files consist of one to eight
characters prefixed by a minus sign "-". The legal characters for
temporary files are the same as those for permanent files.

2. MTS Command Prototype Conventions

For the MTS commands described below, the following
conventions will apply:

    -- Lowercase text represents an item that is to be specified
       by the user.

    -- Uppercase text must be entered verbatim by the user.

    -- Text enclosed in brackets "[]" is optional.

    -- Underlining indicates the minimum abbreviated portion of
       the command that may be used in lieu of the command name
       spelled out in full.

    -- The prefacing of MTS commands with a dollar sign "$" is
       optional in MTS when operating from a terminal. For the
       sake of clarity, the "$" will be included with all MTS
       commands to distinguish MTS commands from ASCS-II
       commands.

3. The MTS $COPY Command

The $COPY command description to follow is presented only for
its usage in the context of ASCS-II operations. In this light
its purpose is to print the contents of a file on the user's
terminal. Its prototype is:

```
$COPY   filename
        -
```

where "filename" is the file specified by the user to be printed
at the user's terminal.
    Note, normally the MTS "PREFIX" switch is set ON. When this
is the case and the $COPY command is executed to print the
contents of a file on the user's terminal, the MTS prefix
character ">" precedes each printed line of output. This prefix
character, like other MTS prefix characters, is an attempt by MTS
to assist the user in interpretation of MTS system activity. If
the user wants the file contents to be printed without the prefix
character, then the MTS "$SET PREFIX=OFF" command should be
issued prior to issuing the $COPY command. Following the
printing of the file's contents, the user is advised to issue the
MTS "$SET PREFIX=ON" command so that prefix characters will once
again appear with the output on the user's terminal. "PFX" is
the MTS abbreviation for "PREFIX."

    4.   The MTS $CREATE Command

    The $CREATE command is used to explicitly create a permanent
or temporary file. The command prototype is:

```
$CREATE   filename   [TYPE=SEQ]
          --
```

 where "filename" is the user-chosen name for the file to be
created.
    If "filename" is preceded by a minus "-" sign, then the file
created will be a temporary file. If "TYPE=SEQ" is included in
the CREATE command, then the file created will be a sequential
file.

Examples:
```
        1)   $CREATE MYFILE
        2)   $CREATE -TEMP
        3)   $CR SFILE TYPE=SEQ
        4)   $CR -TSF TYPE=SEQ
```

    In the first example, a line file named "MYFILE" is created.
In the second example, a temporary line file named "-TEMP" is
created. In the third example, a sequential file named "SFILE"
is created. In the fourth example, a temporary sequential file
named "-TSF" is created.
    Note, if a temporary file does not currently exist and is
part of an MTS command other than $CREATE, $EMPTY, or $DESTROY,
then the temporary file will be implicitly created; i.e., the
first time it is referenced, it will be created.

    5.   The MTS $DESTROY Command

    The $DESTROY command is used to destroy a file (either
permanent or temporary) and its contents. The prototype is:

```
        $DESTROY  filename  [OK]
                  ---
```

where "filename" is the file the user specifies to be destroyed.
     The "OK" is the user's means of confirming that "filename"
is to be destroyed. For temporary files, no confirmation is
required. For permanent files, if the confirmation is not given
with the command, then MTS prompts for it by:

```
     #FILE "filename" IS TO BE DESTROYED.  PLEASE CONFIRM.
     ?
```

A response of "OK" will then destroy the file and a response of
"NO" will cancel the $DESTROY command.

Examples:
     1) $DESTROY ABC OK
     2) $DES -TEMP

     6.   The MTS $EDIT Command

     The $EDIT command is used to invoke the MTS file editor for
the purpose of altering a file's contents. The prototype for the
$EDIT command is:

```
     $EDIT filename
           --
```

 where "filename" is the file specified by the user to be edited.
     There should be little need if any for ASCS-II users to have
to edit a file. If, however, there is a need, then the user is
directed to obtain further instructions on using the editor from
the editor's on-line "EXPLAIN" facility. Simply enter "EXPLAIN"
once in the editor. Following the introductory information that
is printed, the major items that the user is suggested to review
via the editor's EXPLAIN facility are: EDITMODE, LPAR,
COLUMN-RANGES, STRINGS, ALTER, APPEND, COPY, DELETE, INSERT,
MOVE, MTS, OVERPRINT, PRINT, RENUMBER, SCAN, SET, STOP, UNDO,
@ALL, @LINENUMBER, @PRINTCOLUMN, @RIGHTTOLEFT and @VERIFY.

     7.   The MTS $EMPTY Command

     The $EMPTY command is used to empty a file (either permanent
or temporary) of its contents without destroying the file itself.
The prototype is:

```
     $EMPTY  filename  [OK]
             ---
```

where "filename" is the file specified by the user to be emptied.
     The "OK" is the user's means of confirming that "filename"
is to be emptied. For temporary files, no confirmation is
required. For permanent files, if the confirmation is not given
with the command, then MTS prompts for it by:

#FILE "filename" IS TO BE EMPTIED. PLEASE CONFIRM.
 .?

A response of "OK" will then empty the file and a response of "NO" will cancel the $EMPTY command.

Examples:
    1) $EMPTY ABC OK
    2) $EMP -TEMP

    8.   The MTS $LIST Command

    The $LIST command description to follow is presented only for its use in the context of ASCS-II operations. That purpose is to print at the terminal the lines of a file preceded by each line's file linenumber. The prototype is:

    $LIST   filename
         -

where "filename" is the file specified by the user to be printed at the terminal.

Examples:
    1) $LIST MYFILE
    2) $L YOURFILE

    9. The MTS $RENAME Command

    The $RENAME command is used to change the name of a file and/or change a file's status from temporary to permanent or vice versa. The prototype is:

    $RENAME   filename1 filename2 [OK]
    ------

where "filename1" is the name of the file to be changed and "filename2" is the new name for the file.
    If filename1 is the name of a permanent file, then the confirmation of "OK" is required. If confirmation is required and not included with the RENAME command, then MTS prompts the user to confirm by:

    #FILE "filename1" TO BE RENAMED AS "filename2". PLEASE
CONFIRM.
        ?

A response of "OK" will then perform the rename operation and a response of "NO" will cancel the RENAME command.

Examples:
    1) $RENAME MYFILE YOURFILE OK
    2) $RENAME -SS SSSS
    3) $RENAME XXXX -XX OK

In the first example the permanent file "MYFILE" has its name changed to "YOURFILE."   The second example changes the temporary file "-SS" to a permanent file with the name "SSSS." In the third example the permanent file "XXXX" is changed to a temporary file named "-XX."

G.   The ASCS-II Simulator -- General Information

The ASCS-II simulator is an interactive computer program designed to perform the following functions under user control:

1. Construction of an on-line model.
2. Saving a constructed model on off-line disk storage.
3. Retrieval of a model from off-line disk storage and restoring it to an on-line working condition.
4. Model modifications.
5. Setting of program control switches.
6. Adjusting for fixed random number seeds.
7. Model simulation.
8. Printing a description of model structure and parameter settings.
9. Production and display of statistics resulting from model simulation.
10. Production of auxiliary statistics resulting from model simulation. Statistics produced are automatically placed in off-line storage for later analysis.

Since it is not necessary for a user to understand the ASCS-II in depth in order to perform the simulation, only selected aspects of functions 2 through 9 will be presented. Section VIII.H will describe each of the selected ASCS commands and section VIII.I will instruct the user in the resimulation process. The rest of this section will present a variety of topics that should aid the user in understanding the ASCS-II.

1.   The ASCS-II Hospital Admissions Model

ASCS-II is designed so that a wide variety of hospital configurations can be accurately modeled in terms of both the patient flows and the hospital policies governing patient flows. This is accomplished by having a model with three levels of major components that form a hierarchical structure anchored in the model's foundation structure. For all intents and purposes, only its switches are user-changeable. Components for levels one through three, on the other hand, may vary in number, structure, and in their parameter values. Once a model is ready for simulation, all of its components are defined and fixed in number and structure. Therefore, the simulation process only involves adjusting selected model parameters to produce the desired results.

At the first level of the model are the units which correspond one-to-one with those established in the model definition as described by the block diagram (see Chapter VII).

These units represent logical collections of beds within the hospital. Each unit traditionally consists of one or more hospital services or specialty clinics that have been grouped according to attributes they have in common; i.e., levels of care, orientation of care, and proximity of beds.

The second level of the model is devoted to the patient flows into, between, and out of the units. Patient demand for admission is controlled by the four arrival stream components: 1) a.m. emergency, 2) scheduled, 3) call-in and 4) p.m. emergency. These components are the only outside sources of patients for the simulation model.

Upon admission each patient is assigned a length of stay (LOS) based on the LOS distributions (day of the week specific) associated with the patient's particular arrival stream. The LOS assigned is for the patient's initial segment of stay and therefore does not necessarily constitute the patient's entire hospital LOS.

To provide the linkage between each of the patient flow vectors (arrival streams and inter-unit transfers) and their corresponding sets of LOS distributions, second level components called "Input Ports" are used. Upon seeking admission to a unit, a patient is assigned an "Intended Unit" and an "Intended Input Port." The combination of the two identifies the set of LOS distributions to be used in the assignment of LOS for the patient's upcoming segment of stay. The Intended Unit becomes the patient's "Best Unit" for the upcoming segment of stay and the patient is said to "Belong" to this Best Unit for the duration of that segment of stay. Note, the patient may or may not reside on his/her Best Unit depending on that unit's occupancy situation.

With the completion of a segment of stay a patient is either transferred to another unit or discharged from the hospital. To determine which, the set of "Output Port" components (second level) associated with the patient's Best Unit are used. If the patient's Best Unit has no Output Ports, then the patient is discharged. If it has Output Ports, then each designates a next destination (Unit and Input Port) or that the patient be discharged. By sampling a probability distribution associated with the Output Ports, one Output Port is selected and the patient's next destination is determined. The Output Port's destination unit, if discharge is not indicated, then becomes the patient's new Best Unit for the upcoming segment of stay. Note, because the parameter values associated with Output Ports are only changed when a model is totally revised, no further discussion will be devoted to their maintenance.

Alternate Actions constitute the third level components and are used to provide additional means for patients to gain admission to an acceptable unit after first being denied admission to their intended unit. These Alternate Actions make it possible for a patient to 1) gain admission elsewhere on a temporary basis, 2) gain admission elsewhere for the duration of the current segment of stay or 3) force another patient to transfer elsewhere to make a bed available to the incoming patient in his/her intended unit. Any number of Alternate

Actions can be associated with each of the model's Input Ports to be executed in sequence when necessary. In theory, all of the model's patient flows could have their own specific sequence of alternatives, though this is seldom done.

   2. ASCS-II -- Program Start-up

   Since its beginning, ASCS-II has undergone a number of modifications either to accommodate various hospital configurations or simply to refine aspects of its technology. As a result, models constructed under earlier versions may not be compatible with the current version (5.21) of ASCS-II. This does not mean that models incompatible with the ASCS-II version 5.21 cannot still be simulated; their corresponding versions of ASCS-II have been retained and can be made available. Though ASCS-II version 5.21 was brought on-line in December, 1981, another program exists (called ASCS_UPDATE available through the authors) to update any model constructed on ASCS-II version 5.00 or later. This same sort of update capability will be available for all future versions of ASCS-II as well.
   Because of this history of modification to ASCS-II, it is necessary to warn the user that the command to access ASCS-II, given below, is subject to change.
   For ASCS-II version 5.21, the program is initiated by issuing the following MTS command: $SOU TC7B:SIMIT

Upon entering the program, the following text appears and the user is in command mode (indicated by the program prompting message "--CMD:").

     #$SOU TC7B:SIMIT
     #$SET ECHO=OFF
     #EXECUTION BEGINS

     <*><*><*> ASCS SIMULATOR II VERSION(5.21) <*><*><*>

          06/30/82 --   12:01:05

     --CMD:

The date and time appearing after the line with "<*><*><*>" indicates the date and time that ASCS-II is entered.
   Upon ASCS-II program start-up, the user is given 50 seconds of Central Processing Unit (CPU) time to perform work before ASCS-II program execution is suspended. This time limit is necessary in order to prevent a user's funds from being exhausted if a program bug is uncovered during ASCS-II execution. When ASCS-II program suspension occurs in this manner, the following MTS message is printed:

     #LOCAL TIME LIMIT EXCEEDED AT XXXXXXXX

where XXXXXXXX is some program address in ASCS-II and should be ignored by the user.

Assuming that program suspension was not due to a program bug, then program execution can be resumed at the point where suspension occurred by issuing the following MTS restart command:

    $RESTART T=50

or in the abbreviated fashion:

    $RES T=50

Upon reentry to ASCS-II, the user will have another 50 seconds of CPU time for processing. By far the most CPU time-consuming aspect of ASCS-II execution is the simulation itself. Such commands as FETCH, SAVE, CHANGE, XEC, etc. take very little CPU time. As a rule of thumb, about 8 to 12 simulations can be performed in 50 CPU seconds, depending on the length of simulation and the model's total bed complement.

3.   The ASCS-II Fixed Seeds

For the random activities that occur in ASCS-II, the monte-carlo simulation technique is used; i.e., random number generators are used in conjunction with cumulative probability density functions to determine the integer levels associated with the random variables. It is by this technique that such activities as emergency arrival rates, length of stays, and request queues can be modeled and simulated.

At the heart of the random number generators is the "seed," which is a positive, odd integer. As long as the same seed is used to initialize the random number generator at the beginning of every simulation, the resulting stream of random numbers produced by the generator will be the same for every simulation.

In ASCS-II, every aspect of the model depending on random events has its own dedicated random number generator and seed. As a result, some models may have 200 or more generators and seeds. When a simulation is initiated, one seed is picked from which all of the internal model seeds are deterministically set (no two seeds internal to the model will be the same). As long as there is no change in the model's structure, one particular seed must produce the same set of internal model seeds every time.

Via the "SET FIXSEED" command, a particular initial seed can be specified to be used each time the model is simulated, thus giving rise to the term "fixed seed" (see the SET FIXSEED command in this chapter, section VIII.H.7.c). It is to the user's advantage to use a fixed seed. If not, a random initial seed is used and the effects of changing model parameters between simulations may be masked by the uncontrolled variations in the random aspects of the model -- particularly the emergency arrival rates.

4. ASCS-II -- Simulation Rules and Considerations

   Simulation is a two-stage process consisting of a warm-up
stage and a simulation stage. At the outset of the warm-up
stage, all of the model's random number generators are
initialized and all of the model's statistics collection
variables are set to zero. The warm-up stage is completed when
25 weeks have been simulated. At that point, anomalies in unit
censuses should have disappeared and the patient flows should
have stabilized into patterns consistent with the model's
configuration and parameter settings.
   At the conclusion of the warm-up stage, the model's
simulation statistics collection variables are again set to zero
and simulation is performed for the time span specified in the
"SIMULATE" command. Upon concluding the simulation stage,
program control is returned to the user at which time the model
can be queried for averaged result statistics describing the
model's performance during the simulation stage.
   The following is a list of events that occur and in the
order they occur during a simulated day:

   1. UNIT DISCHARGE PROCESSING -- Each unit is checked for
      patients that have completed their segment of length of
      stay and that are to be discharged. These patients are
      now discharged and removed from the model.

   2. UNIT TRANSFER PROCESSING -- Each unit is checked
      according to the "TRANSFER ORDER SPECIFICATIONS" model
      parameters for patients in need of transfer. These
      patients consist of those who have just completed a
      segment of length of stay as well as those whose current
      bed location is unacceptable. An attempt is now made to
      transfer these patients in the same order.

   3. AM RANDOM ARRIVAL PROCESSING -- Each of the model's units
      generate their AM random arrivals (emergencies). The
      order in which each of the model's patients attempt
      admission to the model is randomized.

   4. SCHEDULE STREAM PROCESSING -- According to the "SCHEDULE
      ORDER SPECIFICATIONS," each of the model's unit's
      schedule streams is processed. This processing involves
      first checking how many patients need to be canceled (if
      any), and then admitting the balance of the number
      scheduled.

   5. CALL-IN STREAM PROCESSING -- According to the "CALL-IN
      ORDER SPECIFICATIONS," each of the model's unit's call-in
      streams is processed. If the queue processing option is
      in effect, then:

      a. Requests for the call-in queue are generated and
          added to the queue.

b. Two counts of empty beds available to the call-in stream are made. The first consists of the number of empty beds available to the call-in stream minus the call-in stream's CENSUS REDUCTION ALLOWANCE (CRA). If this number is greater than the stream's CMAX allowance, then it is replaced by the stream's CMAX allowance. The second count consists only of the total number of empty beds that are available to the call-in stream.

c. If the first count is positive, then patients are called in from the queue so that the patients who have been on the queue the greatest number of days are brought in first. The number of patients called in cannot exceed either the first count or the number of patients on the queue. The patients called in by this process are referred to as "REGULAR CALL-INS."

d. If for the remaining patients on the queue, there are patients whose stay on the queue is greater than or equal to the "INTENDED MAXIMUM STAY ON THE QUEUE" parameter, then an attempt is made to bring in these patients as "FORCED CALL-INS." The number of FORCED CALL-INS is limited to the smaller of the second count minus the number of patients already called in (REGULAR) and the number of patients that are in need of a FORCED CALL-IN ADMISSION.

e. Any remaining patients who have stayed on the queue longer than the "ABSOLUTE MAXIMUM STAY ON QUEUE" parameter are then converted into a queue failure statistic.

    If the request queue mechanism is not being used, then an infinite number of patients is available to be called in. Based on this assumption, the number of empty beds available to the call-in stream is compared to the stream's CMAX and CRA and the number of patients to be called in is determined.

6. PM RANDOM ARRIVAL PROCESSING -- Each of the model's units generate their PM random arrivals (emergencies). The order in which each of the model's patients attempt admission to the model is randomized.

7. DAILY STATISTICS PROCESSING -- At the end of the simulated day, statistics are processed prior to beginning the next simulated day.

H.   The ASCS-II Command Language

   · The command language of ASCS-II is designed to minimize user
effort.   In general, it is a free format language with only a few
exceptions.   This means that spacing between keywords and
parameters of the commands is unimportant.

   Upon entering the program, "--CMD: " is the first prompting
message encountered.   This prompt indicates that ASCS-II is in
command mode and is ready to accept a command from one of the
nineteen command types (this chapter will discuss only parts of
nine of the command types needed to resimulate an existing
admissions simulation model).

   For some command types, a submode exists which is invoked by
the keyword for the command type.   Once invoked, subsequent
ASCS-II prompts originate from the submode and consist of the
command type keyword followed by a colon;   e.g., "CHANGE: ",
"DISPLAY: ", etc. This allows the user to issue any subsequent
submode commands without prefacing the command with the command
type keyword.   To execute a command not belonging to the current
submode, the user simply prefaces the command with the keyword
corresponding to the desired command type.

   For those command types not having a submode, the command
keyword invokes the appropriate processing, and ASCS-II then
returns to command mode.   These commands have only one aspect of
processing associated with them and are therefore not repeatedly
invoked.

   Most commands and all submode commands require parameters.
These parameters are of three types: 1) submode keywords, 2)
range parameters indicating locations within the model, and 3)
program control parameters.   If these parameters are entered with
the command, they must appear in the order required by the
command or submode command.   If omitted, ASCS-II will prompt for
them one at a time.   All prompting messages are terminated by a
colon and a space.   In response to any prompt at any level of
processing, the user may enter "STOP" to discontinue the current
command being processed and return to command mode.

   Each of the command types and submode commands presented in
section VIII.H will appear with prototypes, examples, and related
prompting messages.   If a submode for the command type exists,
then the prototype will start with the submode prompting message
(keyword for the submode followed by a colon);   otherwise, the
prototype will start as prompted from command mode.   Following
the prompting message, the rest of the prototype will indicate
the format(s) and order of the user responses.   Items enclosed in
brackets "[]" are optional and need not be entered.   Items
enclosed within braces "{}" represent user choices from which
exactly one item must be selected.   Each choice is separated by a
vertical bar "|".   Underlined items are parameters which may or
may not be included in the response.   If omitted, ASCS-II will
prompt for their values individually.   Each item in a response
must be separated by one or more blanks.   Responses to prompts
requesting ranges may be a single number, two numbers separated
by a hyphen with no embedded blanks, or the word "ALL," implying
the maximum range.

Figure VIII-1 is a description of the abbreviations used both in this chapter and by the ASCS-II program. Any abbreviation preceded by "#" is read as "number of." Following the abbreviation, "#" simply means "number." For example, "#U" and "U#" represent "number of units" and "unit number" respectively.

```
 1. AA          Alternate Action
 2. AM          AM Random Arrival Stream
 3. BU          Best Unit
 4. CAN         Cancellation Allowance
 5. CI          Call-in Stream
 6. CMAX        Call-in Maximum Allowance
 7. CRA         Census Reduction Allowance
 8. CU          Co-Unit
 9. DEST_IP     Destination Input Port
10. DEST_U      Destination Unit
11. DSCB        Daily Statistic Control Block
12. FC          Force Criteria
13. IP          Input Port
14. OP          Output Port
15. PM          PM Random Arrival Stream
16. SC          Schedule/Call-in Arrival Stream
17. SCHED       Schedule Allowance for a Schedule Stream
18. SD          Schedule Stream
19. U           Unit
20. UA          Unit Allowance
```

FIGURE VIII-1 -- Key to ASCS-II Abbreviations

1.   The ASCS-II ADJUST Command

Prototype --

    --CMD: ADJUST [REINIT]

The use of the ADJUST command may be considered an advanced aspect of the simulation strategy. It is used to determine the adjustment factors for each of the random number generators that are used by the random arrival streams and the request queue generators when a fixed seed has been set. The principle behind the adjustment factors is to modify the mean of the numbers produced by the generators so that they approximate the intended means to be produced during simulation.

The need for these adjustment factors is due to the following. Each of the arrival rate distributions, when established for the model, were created based on mean arrival rates supplied by the user. Because the distributions are poisson in nature, the mean of each is the rate "INTENDED" to be produced during simulation. If one of these distributions were randomly sampled an infinite number of times, then the mean of the samples would equal the mean of the distribution. Since during simulation these arrival rate distributions are randomly sampled a fixed number of times (i.e., once for each day of the simulation stage), it is rare for the means of the samples to equal the means of the distributions. Finally, the resulting mean for a fixed number of samples also depends on the initial random number generator seed used in the sampling process; i.e., different initial seeds result in different sample means. By using adjustment factors appropriately set for the initial seed of each of these random number generators, sampling of the distributions is corrected so that differences between the simulated and intended arrival rates is made negligible.

Basically, the adjustment process involves alternating simulation of the model and the execution of the ADJUST command until the model's adjustment factors are properly set. This process normally takes about eight sets of the simulation/adjustment cycles. Because the ADJUST command utilizes an algorithm to home automatically in on the appropriate adjustment factors, it is seldom necessary for the user to do any manual setting of the adjustment factors. During the adjustment portion of the simulation/adjustment cycle, the user can observe the spread between the INTENDED and SIMULATED rates. When the difference between them is negligible for a stream, an indication that the stream's adjustment factor is properly set appears in the right most column of the ADJUST command's output (see Figure VIII-2).

The "REINIT" parameter, when accompanying the ADJUST command, reinitializes the adjustment algorithm and resets all adjustment factors to 1.0. If REINIT does not accompany the ADJUST command, then modifications are made to those adjustment factors whose streams deviate from their intended arrival rates.

The adjustment of random number generators need only be done when: 1) new components are added to the model (this is not within the scope of this chapter), 2) changes to random arrival stream rates have been made in the model or 3) adjustment needs to be done for a different length of simulation or for another fixed seed. The methodology to perform the adjustment process is as follows:

1. With a model on-line, via the SET command, set the FIXSEED "OFF" and the ADJFACT switch "OFF."

2. Select the length of simulation to be used for this model's fixed seed: 100 or 200 weeks.

3. Change all SCHEDULE and CMAX allowances to zero. Set the QFORCE switch to "OFF" if the model has request queue generators. This step will reduce the costs of the adjustment process.

4. Simulate the model for the number of weeks selected in step #2.

5. Via the SET command, set the FIXSEED "ON" and to the seed displayed for the last simulation. Also set the ADJFACT switch "ON."

6. Execute the ADJUST command with the REINIT parameter. This reinitializes the adjustment process algorithm to its starting point.

7. Execute the ADJUST command without the REINIT parameter. This step engages the adjustment process algorithm to compare the SIMULATED weekly rates with the INTENDED weekly rates. When the differences between each of the streams' INTENDED and SIMULATED rates are still significant, the streams' adjustment factors are reset automatically for the next simulation. The automatic setting of the adjustment factors is based on an application of the Central Limit Theorem. After the rate comparison and adjustment factors for each stream have been reset (if necessary), the results of this cycle of the adjustment process are printed (see Figure VIII-2).

8. If all streams appear to be adjusted (the last column titled "DONE" in the ADJUST command output will contain "XXXX" for every stream with an adjustment factor), then go to step #12.

9. If individual adjustment factors appear to be grossly out of adjustment (greater than 300% deviation), then they may be changed manually at this time via the "CHANGE AMADJUST," "CHANGE PMADJUST" or "CHANGE QADJUST" commands. In so doing, the user is overriding the algorithm in the ADJUST command with the intent of homing in on the appropriate adjustment factor sooner.

10. Simulate the model again for the number of weeks selected in step #2.

11. Go to step #7.

12. Use the CHANGE commands to restore the SCHEDULE and CMAX allowances to their desired values. If the model has request queue generators, use the SET command to set the QFORCE switch "ON."

13. Save the adjusted model.

14. The adjustment process is completed.

2. The ASCS-II CHANGE Command

The ASCS-II CHANGE command is used to alter the values of a model's component's parameters. The command has a submode so that the user may change a number of parameters in sequential fashion while entering the keyword "CHANGE" only once at the beginning of the sequence. For this chapter only twenty-one of the CHANGE submode keywords will be presented.

```
--CMD: ADJUST
```

U#	STREAM#	INTENDED RATE TO BE ATTAINED	SIMULATED RATE ATTAINED	PERCENT DEVIATION IN RATES	CURRENT ADJUSTMENT FACTOR	NEW ADJUSTMENT FACTOR	DONE
1	AM#= 1	3.649	3.950	8.249	1.01927	1.00359	
1	PM#= 1	13.498	14.040	4.015	1.01872	1.00587	
2	AM#= 1	0.031	0.070	125.806	1.05500	1.01210	
2	PM#= 1	0.062	0.250	303.225	1.10667	1.01551	
3	AM#= 1	13.402	13.320	-0.612	0.98107	0.98370	
3	PM#= 1	65.653	65.710	0.087	1.00942	1.00942	XXXX
4	AM#= 1	7.404	7.400	-0.054	0.98986	0.98986	XXXX
4	PM#= 1	22.341	22.280	-0.273	0.99601	0.99694	
3	CI#= 1	17.493	17.430	-0.360	0.96813	0.97188	

Figure VIII-2 An Example of Output Produced by the ADJUST
Command During the Middle of the Adjustment Process

a. The AA Keyword of the CHANGE Submode

Prototype --

```
CHANGE: AA   U# RANGE   IP# RANGE   AA# RANGE
        --------  ---------  ---------
```

The AA keyword permits the user to change the ALTERNATE
ACTIONS that are associated with the patient flow vectors
associated with the units. These ALTERNATE ACTIONS, when
present, provide a means for patients to gain admission to a unit
other than their intended unit after first being denied admission
to their intended unit. The patient flow vector (stream) into
the intended unit of admission, providing the ALTERNATE ACTIONS,
is identified by its INPUT PORT NUMBER (IP#). There are four
types of alternate actions:

1. REDIRECTION (specified by "R") -- This alternate action
directs the patient to seek residence on another unit on a
temporary basis; i.e., gain admission to the unit of redirection
and then attempt admission to the patient's intended unit as soon
as a bed becomes available.

2. CO-UNIT REASSIGNMENT (specified by "C") -- This alternate
action directs the patient to seek admission on another unit (the
CO-UNIT) that will be a satisfactory residence for the patient
for the duration of the patient's current segment of stay. The
patient will not attempt to transfer to his/her intended unit
during this segment of stay but will continue to BELONG TO the
intended unit of admission even though not residing there. The
CO-UNIT alternate action can only be specified for those units
that are CO-UNITS of the intended unit of admission.

VIII - 132

Note, in order for a co-unit's beds to be included in the computations that are a part of the decision for cancellations and number of patients to call in, the stream's input port must have a CO-UNIT alternate action specifying the co-unit. For certain situations it is desirable to have the beds included in the computations, but not to have the patients reside on the co-unit on a CO-UNIT basis. To accomplish this, a REDIRECTION alternate action to the co-unit must appear in the input port's set of alternate actions prior to the CO-UNIT alternate action to the co-unit.

   3. FORCE (specified by "F") -- This alternate action attempts to find a patient (called the candidate) in the intended unit of admission who can be safely transferred (forced) into the unit indicated by the FORCE alternate action and reside there for the remainder of the candidate's segment of stay. If such a candidate patient is found and there is a bed available in the unit indicated by the alternate action, then a bed in the intended unit becomes available for the patient causing this FORCE and the alternate action is successful.

   4. SKIP (specified by "SKIP") -- This alternate action is a null alternate action; i.e., the alternate action component is still available in the model but has no effect on simulation.

Example:

```
   CHANGE: AA 1 2-3 ALL
   <*><*>    ALTERNATE ACTION SPECIFICATIONS   <*><*>
   J1) U#   IP#   AA#:  U_DEST#   IP_DEST#   TYPE   #U_SFS   SFS_UNITS
       1     2    1:      2          3        R
       1     2    2:      8          1        R
       1     2    3:
       1     2    4:      4          9        F       3      1  3  4
       1     3    1: 2 3 C
       1     3    2:    SKIP
       1     3    3: 4 5 R
```

where:

   1. U_DEST# specifies the unit in which the patient (or candidate in the case of a FORCE alternate action) is to seek admission.

   2. IP_DEST# specifies the input port through which the patient (or candidate in the case of a FORCE alternate action) is to seek admission into the unit specified by U_DEST#.

   3. TYPE is the alternate action type specification; i.e., R, C, F or SKIP.

4. #U_SFS is used only for the FORCE alternate action. As an acronym, it stands for "the number of units in the selective force screen." Since "3" was entered in the above example, 3 unit numbers appeared in the next field.

5. SFS UNITS specifies the units comprising the SELECTIVE FORCE SCREEN. For a patient to be considered a candidate, the patient must belong to one of the units in this SELECTIVE FORCE SCREEN.

6. Responses to the prompting messages of this CHANGE subcommand are free formatted; i.e., they do not have to be placed under the columns.

7. A null response (simply a carriage return) will result in no change for the alternate action component.

b. The ALLOW Keyword of the CHANGE Submode

Prototype --

        CHANGE: ALLOW U# RANGE SC# RANGE
                       -------- ---------

The ALLOW keyword is used to change all four of the allowances (CAN, CMAX, CRA and SCHED) for a range of SCHEDULE and CALL-IN streams all at once. The ALLOW keyword produces a matrix-prompting sequence which expects a semi-free formatted response to set the values in each of the allowances. This matrix-prompting sequence is also used for each of the following individual CHANGE submode commands: CAN, CMAX, CRA and SCHED. For each of these submode commands, there is a five character window under each day column identifier in which the user may place a response. This window includes the three spaces directly beneath the three character day of the week column title and one space to the left and right of it. Concerning the user's response, if the window contains all blanks, then no change is made to that element of the allowance. If a null response (simply a carriage return) is entered, then no change is made to the allowance vector. For example, the following two sequences produce the same results:

Sequence #1

        CHANGE: ALLOW 2 1
        <*><*>   SCHEDULE/CALLIN SPECIFICATIONS <*><*>
        H3) U#   SC#   ITEM: SUN   MON   TUE   WED   THU   FRI   SAT
             2   1   CAN: 0   0   0   0   0   0   0
             2   1   CMAX:
             2   1   CRA: 31   27   12   9   15
             2   1   SCHED: 2   2   2   2   2

Sequence #2

```
· CHANGE: ALLOW 2 1
  <*><*>   SCHEDULE/CALLIN SPECIFICATIONS  <*><*>
  H3) U#  SC#   ITEM:  SUN  MON  TUE  WED  THU  FRI  SAT
      2    1    CAN:   0         0 0       0    0    0    0
      2    1    CMAX:
      2    1    CRA:        3127            12   9   15
      2    1    SCHED: 2         2 2       2    2
```

    c.   The AMADJUST Keyword of the CHANGE Submode

Prototype --

       CHANGE: AMADJUST U# RANGE AM# RANGE
                      -------- ---------

    The AMADJUST keyword is used to change the adjustment factor for the AM emergency arrival streams. See section VIII.H.1 for more detailed information concerning the purpose and use of adjustment factors.

Example:

```
CHANGE: AMADJUST 1-2 1
<*><*>  AM EMERGENCY ARRIVAL SPECIFICATIONS  <*><*>
ENTER U#=1  AM#=1 ADJUSTMENT FACTOR: 1.00951
ENTER U#=2  AM#=1 ADJUSTMENT FACTOR: 0.99875
```

    d.   The AMDISTS Keyword of the CHANGE Submode

Prototype --

       CHANGE: AMDISTS U# RANGE AM# RANGE
                     -------- ---------

    The AMDISTS keyword is used to change the distributions that are used in the random generation of AM emergency arrivals to the units. For this chapter, only changes made via the ASCS-II internal Poisson distribution generating routine are discussed. Seldom is any other mechanism used to set these emergency arrival distributions.

Using the Example on the Next Page:

    1. By entering "P" in response to the prompt "ENTER DISTRIBUTION TYPE:", the user is invoking the built-in Poisson distribution generator to be used in setting the distributions. Then the user need only enter the appropriate distribution means for each day of the week.

2. If a null response (simply a carriage return) is made when a distribution mean is expected, then no change is made to the current day's distribution already assigned.

3. If the word "ALL" is entered after one or more means have been entered for a particular stream, then the last mean entered will be used for the remaining days of the week as well. Entering "ALL" prior to entering a mean value for an emergency arrival stream will result in an error message and the prompt for the distribution mean for the day will be reissued.

4. If the word "NONE" is entered in response to any prompt for a daily mean, then no change will be made to the currently assigned distributions for that day and the remaining days of the week.

Example:

```
CHANGE: AMDISTS 1-3 ALL
<*><*>   AM EMERGENCY ARRIVAL SPECIFICATIONS   <*><*>
ENTER DISTRIBUTION TYPE: P
     U#    AM#    DAY: MEAN
"P"   1     1     SUN: 2.5
"P"   1     1     MON:
"P"   1     1     TUE: 2.75
"P"   1     1     WED: NONE
"P"   2     1     SUN: 2.0 ALL
"P"   3     1     SUN: 1.357
"P"   3     1     MON: 1.894
"P"   3     1     TUE: .987
"P"   3     1     WED: STOP

--CMD:
```

e.   The BADBEDS Keyword of the CHANGE Submode

Prototype --

```
CHANGE: BADBEDS  U# RANGE
                --------
```

The BADBEDS keyword is used to change the distribution (not day of the week specific) that is associated with each unit for the purpose of temporarily reducing bed capacity due to patients in isolation, beds needing maintenance, etc.

Example:

```
CHANGE: BADBEDS 3
D6) U#= 3 ENTER MEAN # OF UNUSEABLE BEDS:  2.475
```

f. The BMAXCAP Keyword of the CHANGE Submode

Prototype --

    CHANGE: BMAXCAP U# RANGE BU# RANGE
                     -------- ---------

     The BMAXCAP keyword is used to restrict the maximum number
of patients that can reside on the unit who belong to (should be
residing on) another particular unit. For a model with "N"
units, there is a vector of "N" BMAXCAPs associated with each
unit. BMAXCAP(i,j)=X restricts for unit "i" such that "X" is the
maximum number of patients belonging to unit "j" that may reside
on unit "i" at any one time.
     There is one BMAXCAP in each unit's vector of BMAXCAPs for
which this is not true. That BMAXCAP is the one corresponding to
the unit itself and is called the UNIT ALLOWANCE; i.e.,
BMAXCAP(i,j) where i=j. The UNIT ALLOWANCE is the number of beds
that may not be filled by scheduled or call-in patients and
therefore reduces a unit's capacity when calculations are made
for cancellations and call-ins.

Examples:

    CHANGE: BMAXCAP 2-3 1-3
    <*><*> BMAXCAP SPECIFICATIONS <*><*>
    D6) U# BU#: BMAXCAP
        2   1:
        2   2: 3
        2   3: 45
        3   1: 20
        3   2: 20
        3   3:

and

    CHANGE BMAXCAP 2-3 1-3
    <*><*> BMAXCAP SPECIFICATIONS <*><*>
    D6) U# BU#: BMAXCAP
        2   1: 45 3 45 20 20 0

     In the first example, the change is made one item at a time.
The second example shows that a whole vector of BMAXCAPs and the
UNIT ALLOWANCEs can be changed all at once; though by this
method, all values for the vectors must be entered. In both the
first and second example, the second unit's UNIT ALLOWANCE is set
to 3. In the first example, no change is made to the third
unit's UNIT ALLOWANCE; whereas, in the second example the third
unit's UNIT ALLOWANCE is set to zero.

    g. The CAN Keyword of the CHANGE Submode

Prototype --

        CHANGE: CAN U# RANGE SC# RANGE
                    --------   ---------

        The CAN keyword is used to change the CANCELLATION
ALLOWANCEs associated with the schedule streams in the model.
The cancellation allowance of each schedule stream is used in the
determination of how many of the stream's scheduled patients need
to be cancelled, if any. More specifically, the number specified
by the cancellation allowance represents the number of empty beds
that must be available on the schedule stream's unit and co-units
(as specified by the alternate actions of the input port
associated with the schedule stream) following the admission of
scheduled patients by the schedule stream.

Example:

    CHANGE: CAN 3-4 1
    <*><*>   SCHEDULE/CALLIN SPECIFICATIONS <*><*>
    H7) U#   SC#   ITEM: SUN MON TUE WED THU FRI SAT
         3   1   CAN: 10   8   5   3   0   0   0
         4   1   CAN: 8   4   0

        See the ALLOW CHANGE (see section VIII.H.2.b.) subcommand
concerning this matrix-prompting sequence.

        h. The CAP Keyword of the CHANGE Submode

Prototype --

        CHANGE: CAP U# RANGE

        The CAP keyword is used to change the capacities of the
units in the model. When changing a unit capacity, be sure to
make changes to the unit's BMAXCAP and NBMAXCAP unit parameters
as well if necessary. Example:

    CHANGE: CAP 4
    D1) U#= 4 ENTER CAPACITY: 154

        i. The CMAX Keyword of the CHANGE Submode

Prototype --

        CHANGE: CMAX U# RANGE SC# RANGE
                     --------   ---------

        The CMAX keyword is used to change the CALL-IN MAXIMUM
ALLOWANCEs associated with the call-in streams in the model. The
call-in maximum allowance represents the maximum number of

patients that can be called in to the hospital on a REGULAR basis, as opposed to a FORCED basis for the associated stream, (see section VIII.G.4).

Example:

```
CHANGE: CMAX 3-4 1
<*><*>   SCHEDULE/CALLIN SPECIFICATIONS   <*><*>
H7) U#   SC#   ITEM:   SUN   MON   TUE   WED   THU   FRI   SAT
     3    1    CMAX:    5     5     5     5     5     3     2
     4    1    CMAX:    2     2     2     2     1
```

See the ALLOW CHANGE (see section VIII.H.2.b.) subcommand concerning this matrix-prompting sequence.

j. The CRA Keyword of the CHANGE Submode

Prototype --

```
CHANGE: CRA   U# RANGE   SC# RANGE
              --------   ---------
```

The CRA keyword is used to change the CENSUS REDUCTION ALLOWANCEs associated with the call-in streams in the model. The census reduction allowance (CRA) of each call-in stream is used in the calculations to determine the number of patients that may be safely called in (REGULAR call-ins, see section VIII.G.4.) without causing emergency turnaways or cancellations later in the week. More specifically, the number specified by the CRA represents the number of empty beds after patients have been called in that must be available on the call-in stream's unit and co-units as specified by the alternate actions of the input port associated with the call-in stream.

Example:

```
CHANGE: CRA 1-2 1
<*><*>   SCHEDULE/CALLIN SPECIFICATIONS   <*><*>
H7) U#   SC#   ITEM:   SUN   MON   TUE   WED   THU   FRI   SAT
     1    1    CRA:     50    45    40    41    37    55    79
     2    1    CRA:           40    41    37    55    79
```

See the ALLOW CHANGE (see section VIII.H.2.b.) subcommand concerning this matrix-prompting sequence.

k. The MODEL# Keyword of the CHANGE Submode

Prototype --

```
CHANGE: MODEL#
```

The MODEL# keyword is used to change the number associated with the model. This number is for descriptive or catalogue purposes only and has no effect on simulation outcome.

Example:

    CHANGE: MODEL#
    R1) ENTER NEW MODEL#: 8105

        l. The MOD_DESC Keyword of the CHANGE Submode

Prototype --

    CHANGE: MOD_DESC

The MOD_DESC keyword is used to change the 24 character description associated with the model. It has no effect on simulation outcome.

Example:

    CHANGE: MOD_DESC
    R3) ENTER NEW MODEL DESCRIPTION: GEN. HOSP. FINAL MODEL

        m. The NBMAXCAP Keyword of the CHANGE Submode

Prototype --

    CHANGE: NBMAXCAP   U# RANGE

The NBMAXCAP keyword allows the user to change the unit parameter that restricts the total number of off-service patients on a unit (patients not belonging to the unit). Whereas the BMAXCAP discriminates on a basis of the individual units that the patients belong to, the NBMAXCAP pertains to all patients not belonging to the unit. A unit's BMAXCAP values, excepting the UNIT ALLOWANCE, may not exceed the NBMAXCAP.

Example:

    CHANGE: NBMAXCAP 5
    D5) U#= 5 ENTER MAX CAP FOR NON-BELONGING PATIENTS: 22

        n. The ORDERCI Keyword of the CHANGE Submode

Prototype --

    CHANGE: ORDERCI   ORDER# RANGE

The ORDERCI keyword is used to change the order in which the call-in streams are processed during simulation. When using the

ORDERCI command, it is advisable always to use the "ALL" ORDER#
RANGE since it is unusual to change the order for two streams
adjacent in order.

Example:

```
   CHANGE: ORDERCI ALL
   <*><*>  CALLIN ORDER SPECIFICATIONS  <*><*>
  M1) ORDER#: U#  CI#

          1  :  3      1
          2  :  2      1
          3  :  4      1
          4  :  3      2
```

where:

1. ORDER# -- The position in the stream processing
    sequence.
2. U# -- The intended unit for the call-in stream's
    patients.
3. CI# -- The call-in stream number for the unit.

        o.   The ORDERSD Keyword of the CHANGE Submode

Prototype --

        CHANGE: ORDERSD ORDER# RANGE

     The ORDERSD keyword is used to change the order in which the
schedule streams are processed during simulation.   When using
the ORDERSD command, it is advisable always to use the "ALL"
ORDER# RANGE since it is unusual to change the order for two
streams adjacent in order.

Example:

```
   CHANGE: ORDERSD ALL
   <*><*>   SCHEDULE ORDER SPECIFICATIONS   <*><*>
    M2) ORDER#: U#   SD#
          1  :  3      2
          2  :  4      1
          3  :  2      1
          4  :  3      1
```

where:

1. ORDER# -- The position in the stream-processing sequence.
2. U# -- The intended unit for the schedule stream's
    patients.

    3. SD# -- The schedule stream number for the unit.

    p. The PMADJUST Keyword of the CHANGE Submode

Prototype --

    CHANGE: PMADJUST   U# RANGE   PM# RANGE
                       --------   ---------

    The PMADJUST keyword is used to change the adjustment factor
for the PM emergency arrival streams. See section VIII.H.1. for
more detailed information concerning the purpose and use of
adjustment factors.

Example:

    CHANGE: PMADJUST 1-2 1
    ENTER U#=1 PM#=1 ADJUSTMENT FACTOR: 1.01005
    ENTER U#=2 PM#=1 ADJUSTMENT FACTOR: 0.98238

    q. The PMDISTS Keyword of the CHANGE Submode

Prototype --

    CHANGE: PMDISTS   U# RANGE   PM# RANGE
                      --------   ---------

    The PMDISTS keyword is used to change the distributions that
are used in the random generation of PM emergency arrivals to the
units. For this chapter, only changes made via the ASCS-II
internal Poisson distribution generating routine are discussed.
Seldom is any other mechanism used to set these emergency arrival
distributions.

Example:

    CHANGE: PMDISTS 1-3 ALL
    <*><*>   PM EMERGENCY ARRIVAL SPECIFICATIONS   <*><*>
    ENTER DISTRIBUTION TYPE: P
         U# AM# DAY: MEAN
    "P" 1   1   SUN: 5.4
    "P" 1   1   MON:
    "P" 1   1   TUE: 6.3
    "P" 1   1   WED: ALL
    "P" 2   1   SUN: 4.0 ALL
    "P" 3   1   SUN: 4.775
    "P" 3   1   MON: 5.392
    "P" 3   1   TUE: 3.201
    "P" 3   1   WED: NONE

where:

1. By entering "P" in response to the prompt "ENTER DISTRIBUTION TYPE:", the user is invoking the built-in Poisson distribution generator to be used in setting the distributions. Then the user need only enter the appropriate distribution means for each day of the week.

2. If a null response (simply a carriage return) is made when a distribution mean is expected, then no change is made to the current day's distribution already assigned.

3. If the word "ALL" is entered after one or more means have been entered for a particular stream, then the last mean entered will be used for the remaining days of the week as well. Entering "ALL" prior to entering a mean value for an emergency arrival stream will result in an error message, and the prompt for the distribution mean for the day will be reissued.

4. If the word "NONE" is entered in response to any prompt for a daily mean, then no change will be made to the currently assigned distributions for that day and the remaining days of the week.

   r.   The QADJUST Keyword of the CHANGE Submode

Prototype --

     CHANGE: QADJUST   U# RANGE   SC# RANGE
                       --------   ---------

     The QADJUST keyword is used to change the adjustment factor for the call-in queue generators. See Section VIII.H.1. for more detailed information concerning the purpose and use of adjustment factors.

Example:

     CHANGE: QADJUST 3-4 1
     <*><*> CALLIN QUEUE MONITOR SPECIFICATIONS <*><*>
     U#= 3   SC#= 1   ENTER QUEUE ADJUSTMENT FACTOR: 1.00925
     U#= 4   SC#= 1   ENTER QUEUE ADJUSTMENT FACTOR: 1.01055

   s.   The QDISTS Keyword of the CHANGE Submode

Prototype --

     CHANGE: QDISTS   U# RANGE   SC# RANGE
                      --------   ---------

The QDISTS keyword is used to change the day of the week specific distributions for the call-in queue request generators. In this chapter, only changes made via the ASCS-II internal Poisson distribution generating routine are discussed.

Example:

```
CHANGE: QDISTS 3 1
<*><*>   CALLIN QUEUE MONITOR SPECIFICATIONS  <*><*>
ENTER DISTRIBUTION TYPE: P
     U#  SC#  DAY: MEAN
"P"   3    1  MON: 1.35
"P"   3    1  TUE: 1.45
"P"   3    1  WED:
"P"   3    1  THU: 1.45
"P"   3    1  FRI: ALL
```

where:

1. By entering "P" in response to the prompt "ENTER DISTRIBUTION TYPE:", the user is invoking the built-in Poisson distribution generator to be used in setting the distributions. Then the user need only enter the appropriate distribution means for each day of the week.

2. If a null response (simply a carriage return) is made when a distribution mean is expected, then no change is made to the current day's distribution already assigned.

3. If the word "ALL" is entered after one or more means have been entered for a particular stream, then the last mean entered will be used for the remaining days of the week as well. Entering "ALL" prior to entering a mean value for an emergency arrival stream will result in an error message and the prompt for the distribution mean for the day will be reissued.

4. If the word "NONE" is entered in response to any prompt for a daily mean, then no change will be made to the currently assigned distributions for that day and the remaining days of the week.

   t. The QUEUE Keyword of the CHANGE Submode

Prototype --

     CHANGE: QUEUE U# RANGE SC# RANGE
                    -------- ---------

The QUEUE keyword is used to change both the day of the week specific distributions and the "INTENDED MAXIMUM STAY ON QUEUE" parameters for the call-in queue request generators. For an explanation of the portion of this command concerning the distributions, see the CHANGE QDISTS subcommand. The value assigned to the INTENDED MAXIMUM STAY ON QUEUE is the last day on the queue that a patient can be called in as a REGULAR call-in patient. After the INTENDED MAXIMUM STAY ON QUEUE is passed, every attempt is made to call-in the patient on a FORCED basis; i.e., call the patient in as soon as a bed is available on the unit or its co-units as specified by the alternate actions associated with the call-in stream's input port.

Example:

```
CHANGE: QUEUE 3 1
<*><*> CALLIN QUEUE MONITOR SPECIFICATIONS <*><*>
U#= 3   SC#=1   ENTER INTENDED MAXIMUM STAY ON QUEUE: 3

QUEUE REQUEST DISTRIBUTIONS
ENTER DISTRIBUTION TYPE: P
     U#   SC#   DAY: MEAN
"P"  3     1    SUN: 1.5 ALL
```

u. The SCHED Keyword of the CHANGE Submode

Prototype --

```
CHANGE: SCHED   U# RANGE   SC# RANGE
                --------   ---------
```

The SCHED keyword is used to change the SCHEDULE ALLOWANCE for the schedule streams in the model. This SCHEDULE ALLOWANCE is the day of the week specific numbers of patients that are given fixed dates of admission for the future.

Example:

```
CHANGE: SCHED 3-4 1
<*><*>   SCHEDULE/CALLIN SPECIFICATIONS <*><*>
H7) U#   SC#    ITEM:  SUN  MON  TUE  WED  THU  FRI  SAT
     3    1    SCHED:   15   13   12   11   10    0    0
     4    1    SCHED:    5    5    4    4    3
```

See the ALLOW CHANGE (section VIII.H.2.b.) subcommand concerning this matrix-prompting sequence.

3. The ASCS-II DISPLAY Command

The ASCS-II DISPLAY command is used to display a model's component structure and component parameter values used in simulation. It is also used to display various program switches that govern the ASCS-II program. Like the CHANGE command, the DISPLAY command has a submode that permits the display of various items one after another while entering the keyword "DISPLAY" only once at the beginning of the sequence.

In this chapter, only eighteen of the DISPLAY submode keywords are presented. Generally, the DISPLAY keywords have their counterparts in the CHANGE commands in which the model component and its parameter settings are described in detail. Therefore, if there is a corresponding section in the CHANGE command, then the user is directed to see that section for the more detailed explanation of the particular model component.

    a. The AA Keyword of the DISPLAY Submode

Prototype --

      DISPLAY: AA U# RANGE IP# RANGE AA# RANGE
               -------- --------- ---------

    The AA keyword is used to display the ALTERNATE ACTIONS associated with the model's input ports. The AA keyword of the CHANGE command (see section VIII.H.2.a.) describes the alternate action component's use and parameter settings. The DISPLAY of the alternate actions, however, has a column titled "U_SFS/F_TAG" which is essentially the same as the column "SFS_UNITS" in the CHANGE command description for AA.

Example:

      DISPLAY: AA 1 2-3 ALL

<*><*>   ALTERNATE ACTION SPECIFICATIONS   <*><*>
    U# IP# AA# --TYPE--- U_DEST#   IP_DEST# U_SFS/F_TAG
     1   2   1   F   2   4   1 2 3 4 5 6 7 8
     1   2   2   R   10   1
     1   3   1   C   4   8

    b. The ALLOW Keyword of the DISPLAY Submode.

Prototype --

      DISPLAY: ALLOW U# RANGE SC# RANGE
                      -------- ---------

    The ALLOW keyword is used to display all four of the allowances (CAN, CMAX, CRA and SCHED) for a range of SCHEDULE and CALL-IN streams all at once. See the individual CHANGE keyword subcommands for CAN, CMAX, CRA and SCHED for an explanation of the purpose and use of these allowances.

Example:

```
DISPLAY: ALLOW 3-4 1

<*><*>  ALLOW SPECIFICATIONS  <*><*>
   U#  SC#  ITEM |  SUN  MON  TUE  WED  THU  FRI  SAT
    3    1   CAN  |    0    0    0    0    0    0    0
         1   CMAX |    8    8    8    8    7    5    5
         1   CRA  |   50   45   41   38   35   54   82
         1   SCHED|   15   14   13   12   11    0    0
    4    1   CAN  |    0    0    0    0    0    0    0
         1   CMAX |   99   99   99   99   99    5    5
         1   CRA  |   50   45   41   38   35   54   82
         1   SCHED|    5    4    4    3    3    0    0
```

    c. The AM Keyword of the DISPLAY Submode

Prototype --

    DISPLAY: AM U# RANGE AM# RANGE
                 -------- ---------

The AM keyword is used to display all information contained in the model's AM emergency stream components.

Example:

```
DISPLAY:  AM 6-7 1
<*><*>  AM EMERGENCY SPECIFICATIONS   <*><*>
               DEST.  ADM. INITIAL ADJUST.
U#  AM#   IP#   TYPE   TAG  FACTOR    DIST#   MEAN   VARIANCE   DAYS
 6   1     6     0     111  0.9905     30    1.000    1.004    SUN--MON
                                       31    1.311    1.302    TUE
                                       32    1.031    1.032    WED
                                       24    0.625    0.622    THU
                                       33    1.593    1.585    FRI
                                       34    0.844    0.844    SAT
```

7 HAS NO "AM" EMERGENCY ARRIVALS

where:

    1. U# -- Unit number.

    2. AM# -- AM emergency stream number.

    3. DEST. IP# -- Input port to be used in seeking admission to the destination unit.

    4. ADM. TYPE -- This column may be ignored. It is used only in special analysis situations.

    5. INITIAL TAG -- This column may be ignored. It is used only in special analysis situations.

6. ADJUST. FACT -- Adjustment factor for the AM emergency arrival stream (see section VIII.H.1.).

7. DIST# -- Distribution number. This column is for internal program control and may be ignored.

8. MEAN -- This column displays the mean of the day's arrival distribution. The values displayed may differ slightly from the values entered via the CHANGE AMDISTS subcommand due to truncation.

9. VARIANCE -- This column displays the variance of the day's AM emergency distribution.

10. DAYS -- This column indicates the day(s) of the week for which the distribution is associated.

    d.   The BMAXCAP Keyword of the DISPLAY Submode

Prototype --

     DISPLAY: BMAXCAP U# RANGE   BU# RANGE
                       --------   ---------

     The BMAXCAP keyword is used to display the model's BMAXCAP and UNIT ALLOWANCE values (see the BMAXCAP keyword of the CHANGE subcommand for an explanation of BMAXCAP and UNIT ALLOWANCE, section VIII.H.2.f.).

Example:

     DISPLAY BMAXCAP 3-6 3-6

     <*><*>   BMAXCAP SPECIFICATIONS   <*><*>
          | BESTUNIT NUMBERS
U#	3 4 5 6
3	0 120 120 120
4	138 0 138 138
5	20 20 3 20
6	7 7 7 2

    e.   The CAN Keyword of the DISPLAY Submode

Prototype --

     DISPLAY: CAN U# RANGE   SC# RANGE
                   --------   ---------

The CAN keyword is used to display the CANCELLATION ALLOWANCE (CAN) for the schedule streams. See the CAN CHANGE subcommand for an explanation of the cancellation allowance.

Example:

```
DISPLAY: CAN 3-4 1

<*><*>   CAN SPECIFICATIONS  <*><*>
   U#  SC#  ITEM | SUN  MON  TUE  WED  THU  FRI  SAT
   3    1   CAN  |  12   10    8    6    4    0    0
   4    1   CAN  |   0    0    0    0    0    0    0
```

f. The CMAX Keyword of the DISPLAY Submode.

Prototype --

```
DISPLAY: CMAX  U# RANGE  SC# RANGE
               --------  ---------
```

The CMAX keyword is used to display the CALL-IN MAXIMUM ALLOWANCE (CMAX) for the call-in streams. See the CMAX CHANGE subcommand for an explanation of the call-in maximum allowance.

Example:

```
DISPLAY: CMAX 3-4 1

<*><*>   CMAX SPECIFICATIONS  <*><*>
   U#  SC#  ITEM | SUN  MON  TUE  WED  THU  FRI  SAT
   3    1   CMAX |   8    8    8    8    7    3    3
   4    1   CMAX |   3    3    3    3    3    2    1
```

g. The CRA Keyword of the DISPLAY Submode.

Prototype --

```
DISPLAY: CRA  U# RANGE  SC# RANGE
              --------  ---------
```

The CRA keyword is used to display the CENSUS REDUCTION ALLOWANCE (CRA) for the call-in streams. See the CRA CHANGE subcommand for an explanation of the census reduction allowance.

Example:

```
DISPLAY: CRA 3-4 1

<*><*>   CRA SPECIFICATIONS  <*><*>
   U#  SC#  ITEM | SUN  MON  TUE  WED  THU  FRI  SAT
   3    1   CRA  |  55   48   42   38   35   60   84
   4    1   CRA  |  45   38   32   28   25   50   74
```

h. The IP Keyword of the DISPLAY Submode.

Prototype --

    DISPLAY: IP U# RANGE IP# RANGE
             -------- ---------

    The IP keyword is used to display the INPUT PORTS associated
with the model's units. Of particular interest in this display
is the means of the length of stay distributions. In some cases
during simulation, excessive call-ins on a day with a high mean
length of stay relative to the length of stays for the rest of
the week result in low total rates of admission yet adequate
average daily census. Instructions for changing the length of
stay distributions for input ports is beyond the scope of this
chapter.

Example:

    DISPLAY: IP 3 2

<*><*>	INPUT	PORT	SPECIFICATIONS	<*><*>			
U#	#IP	IP#	AA	MINIMUM TAG	DIST#	MEAN	VARIANCE	DAYS
3	6	2	YES	111	137	13.073	385.884	SUN
					138	13.703	705.331	MON
					139	10.731	104.003	TUE
					140	11.059	74.984	WED
					141	13.207	87.202	THU
					142	11.939	58.389	FRI
					143	14.177	126.824	SAT

where:

    1. U# -- Unit Number.

    2. #IP -- Number of input ports associated with the unit.

    3. IP# -- The number of the input port currently being
       displayed.

    4. AA -- A "YES" or "NO" indication as to whether or not
       the input port has any alternate actions.

5. MINIMUM_TAG -- This column may be ignored. It is used only in special analysis situations.

6. DIST# -- Distribution number. This column is for internal program control and may be ignored.

7. MEAN -- This column displays the mean of the day's length of stay distribution.

8. VARIANCE -- This column displays the variance of the day's length of stay distribution.

9. DAYS -- This column indicates the day(s) of the week for which the distribution is associated.

    i.   The MODEL Keyword of the DISPLAY Submode.

Prototype --

    DISPLAY: MODEL

The MODEL keyword is used to display an entire model via this single command. If a "SET PRINT..." command (see section VIII.H.7.d.) has been previously issued and the "PRINT" switch is in the "ON" position, then the model display will be placed in the disk file specified in the "SET PRINT ..." command. This is the only DISPLAY submode command for which this occurs. It is sometimes handy to display the model in this manner when the model's simulation output and display of the model are to be printed at a remote printer.

Example:

    DISPLAY: MODEL
          .
          .
          .

    j.   The MODEL# Keyword of the DISPLAY Submode.

Prototype --

    DISPLAY: MODEL#

The MODEL# keyword is used to display the model's model number. The model number serves no purpose other than description and cataloguing.

Example:

    DISPLAY: MODEL#

    MODEL #= 905

    K. MOD_DESC keyword of the DISPLAY Submode.

Prototype --

    DISPLAY: MOD_DESC

The MOD_DESC keyword is used to display the 24 character
description that has been given to the model via the MOD_DESC
CHANGE subcommand.

Example:

    DISPLAY: MOD_DESC

    <*><*> GEN. HOSP. FINAL MODEL   <*><*>

    l. The ORDERCI Keyword of the DISPLAY Submode.

Prototype --

    DISPLAY: ORDERCI ORDER# RANGE

The ORDERCI keyword is used to display the order of the
processing of the call-in streams during simulation.

Example:

    DISPLAY: ORDERCI ALL

    <*><*> CALLIN ORDER <*><*>
     ORDER# U# CI# CALLIN_IP#
        1   4   1   2
        2   5   1   2
        3   3   1   8
        4   7   1   2

where:

    1. ORDER# -- The number indicating the position in the processing
       sequence.

    2. U# -- The number of the intended unit into which the call-in
       stream is generating admissions.

VIII - 152

3. CI# -- The call-in stream number for the unit.

4. CALLIN_IP# -- The number of the input port through which the call-in stream is generating its admissions.

   m.   The ORDERSD Keyword of the DISPLAY Submode

Prototype --

    DISPLAY: ORDERSD ORDER# RANGE

The ORDERSD keyword is used to display the order of the processing of the schedule streams during simulation.

Example:

    DISPLAY: ORDERSD ALL

    <*><*>   SCHEDULE ORDER <*><*>
     ORDER# U#   SD#   SCHED_IP#
        1   4   1   3
        2   5   1   2
        3   3   1   7

where:

1. ORDER# -- The number indicating the position in the processing sequence.

2. U# -- The number of the intended unit into which the schedule stream is generating admissions.

3. SD# -- The schedule stream number for the unit.

4. SCHED_IP# -- The number of the input port through which the schedule stream is generating its admissions.

   n.   The PM Keyword of the DISPLAY Submode

Prototype --

    DISPLAY: PM U# RANGE PM# RANGE
                 -------- ---------

The PM keyword is used to display all information contained in the model's PM emergency stream components.

Example:

```
DISPLAY: PM 1-2 ALL

<*><*>  PM EMERGENCY SPECIFICATIONS  <*><*>
              DEST.  ADM.  INITIAL  ADJUST.
  U#   PM#    IP#    TYPE   TAG     FACTOR    DIST#    MEAN    VARIANCE   DAYS
  1     1      1      0     111     1.0057     44     1.967     1.962     SUN
                                               45     2.156     2.156     MON
                                               46     1.749     1.742     TUE
                                               47     1.875     1.869     WED
                                               46     1.749     1.742     THU
                                               48     2.001     2.003     FRI--SAT
  2     1      2      0     111     1.0080      1     0.000     0.000     SUN--MON
                                               16     0.031     0.030     TUE--WED
                                                1     0.000     0.000     THU--SAT
```

where:

1. U# -- Unit number.

2. PM# -- PM emergency stream number.

3. DEST. IP# -- Input port to be used in seeking admission to the destination unit.

4. ADM. TYPE -- This column may be ignored. It is used only in special analysis situations.

5. INITIAL TAG -- This column may be ignored. It is used only in special analysis situations.

6. ADJUST. FACTOR -- Adjustment factor for the PM emergency arrival stream -- see section VIII.H.1.

7. DIST# -- Distribution number. This column is for internal program control and may be ignored.

8. MEAN -- This column displays the mean of the day's arrival distribution. The values displayed may differ slightly from the values entered via the CHANGE PMDISTS subcommand due to truncation.

9. VARIANCE -- This column displays the variance of the day's PM emergency distribution.

10. DAYS -- This column indicates the day(s) of the week for which the distribution is associated.

   o. The QUEUE Keyword of the DISPLAY Submode.

Prototype --

    DISPLAY: QUEUE U# RANGE SC# RANGE
             -------- ---------

    The QUEUE keyword is used to display all of the parameter
values associated with the call-in request queue generators.

Example:

    DISPLAY: QUEUE 3 1

    <*><*> QUEUE MONITOR SPECIFICATIONS <*><*>

    MAXIMUM STAY ON QUEUE= 5
    INTENDED MAXIMUM STAY ON QUEUE= 3 DAYS
    QUEUE ADJUSTMENT FACTOR =   0.99871
    AVERAGE DAILY REQUEST RATE FOR PLACEMENT ON QUEUE
     U# CI#   DIST#   MEAN   VARIANCE DAYS
      3   1   409   1.349   1.344 SUN-SAT

where:

    1. MAXIMUM STAY ON QUEUE -- If a patient remains on the
       queue for the MAXIMUM STAY ON QUEUE value, then the
       patient is turned into a QUEUE FAILURE statistic and is
       removed from the queue (see section VIII.G.5.e.). The
       QUEUE FAILURE statistic should only occur during
       simulation when the number of requests generated are too
       great for the unit (model) to handle.

    2. INTENDED MAXIMUM STAY ON QUEUE -- This parameter
       represents the maximum number of days that a patient may
       wait after requesting admission before gaining admission
       to the hospital. Patients called in from the request
       queue on or before this INTENDED maximum stay on queue
       may only be called in on a REGULAR basis. On or after
       the INTENDED maximum stay on queue patients may be called
       in on either a FORCED or REGULAR basis (see section
       VIII.G.5.e.). This parameter must always be less than or
       equal to the "MAXIMUM STAY ON QUEUE" parameter.

    3. QUEUE ADJUSTMENT FACTOR -- The random number generator
       adjustment factor dedicated to the individual queue (see
       section VIII.H.1.).

    4. U# -- The unit number associated with the queue.

    5. CI# -- The call-in stream number associated with the
       queue.

    6. DIST# -- Distribution number. This column is for
       internal program control and may be ignored.

7. MEAN -- This column displays the mean of the day's request distribution. The values may differ slightly from the values entered via the CHANGE QDISTS subcommand due to truncation.

8. VARIANCE -- This column displays the variance of the day's request distribution.

9. DAYS -- This column indicates the day(s) of the week for which the distribution is associated.

p. The SCHED Keyword of the DISPLAY Submode

Prototype --

    DISPLAY: SCHED U# RANGE SC# RANGE
                    -------- ---------

    The SCHED keyword is used to display the SCHEDULE ALLOWANCE (SCHED) for the model's schedule streams. See the SCHED keyword of the CHANGE subcommand for an explanation of the schedule allowance.

Example:

    DISPLAY: SCHED 3-4 1

    <*><*>   SCHED SPECIFICATIONS   <*><*>
     U# SC# ITEM | SUN MON TUE WED THU FRI SAT
      3   1 SCHED | 8   7   7   7   5   0   0
      4   1 SCHED | 3   3   3   3   2   2   1

    q. The SWITCHES Keyword of the DISPLAY Submode.

Prototype --

    DISPLAY: SWITCHES

    The SWITCHES keyword is used to display the switch settings that are currently in effect that affect the ASCS-II operation. Of these switches, simulation by the engineer will involve most the following four switches:

1. AVG&TOT -- This switch controls the columnar simulation output (see the "XEC" command). In the "ON" position, the output will contain columns for both weekly totals and weekly averages where appropriate. This output, however, may cause problems for those people with terminals having only 80-column-wide output capabilities.

2. DISBEST -- This switch controls the collection of the statistics for discharges from the units during simulation. If in the "ON" position, then statistics reporting discharges from the individual units of the model reflect the discharges of patients who belonged to the individual unit at the time of discharge. As such, the discharge statistics do not necessarily reflect the unit of residence of the patients discharged. In the "OFF" position, the discharge statistics for individual units reflect only the volume of patients discharged from those individual units on the basis of physical location and do not reflect the unit on which patients should have been residing at the time of discharge.

3. QFORCE -- This switch, in the "ON" position, invokes the QUEUE FORCE call-in processing. If in the "OFF" position, only REGULAR CALL-IN processing occurs.

4. ADJFACT -- This switch controls whether or not the ADJUSTMENT FACTORS for the emergency arrival streams and queue request generators are to be used to produce the intended number of arrivals or requests for their streams. In the "ON" position, the adjustment factors are functioning. See section VIII.H.1. for the purpose of the ADJUSTMENT FACTORS.

Example:


```
DISPLAY: SWITCHES

<*><*>  MODEL CONTROL SWITCHES  <*><*>
MIX AM      ON    AM PROCESS MIXING
MIX PM      ON    PM PROCESS MIXING
MIX SD      OFF   SCHEDULE PROCESS MIXING
MIX CI      OFF   CALLIN PROCESS MIXING
AUXSTAT     OFF   AUXILIARY STATISTICS COLLECTION
DOSPD       OFF   DAY-OF-STAY BY PATIENT DAY STATISTICS COLLECTION
DOSPDBYBU   OFF   DAY-OF-STAY STATISTICS TO BE BASED ON BESTUNIT
AVG&TOT     ON    RESULTS COMMAND PRODUCES BOTH AVG. & TOT. COLUMNS
ANTTRANS    OFF   STATISTICS COLLECTED FOR ANTICIPATED TRANSFERS
ALLTRANS    OFF   STATISTICS COLLECTED FOR ALL TRANSFERS
DISBEST     ON    STATISTICS COLLECTED FOR DISCHARGE BY BESTUNIT
QFORCE      ON    QUEUE FORCED CALLINS OPERATIONAL
ADJFACT     ON    ADJUSTMENT FACTORS OPERATIONAL
```

r. The UNIT Keyword of the DISPLAY Submode

Prototype --

DISPLAY: UNIT U# RANGE

    The UNIT keyword is used to display a number of the
parameter settings as well as the number of various components
associated with the model's units.

Example:

    DISPLAY: UNIT 1-4

    <*><*> UNIT SPECIFICATIONS <*><*>
    U# UCBDESC U_TYPE CAP FC NBCAP UA #CU #AM #PM #SC #IF #OP BBEDS
     1 ICU/CCU LIM2   18   1   18   7   0   1   1   0   8   8 0.000
     2 SPCU   REG   22   1   22   0   0   1   1   0   4   2 0.060
     3 MED   REG   151   1   151   0   7   1   1   1   6   6 6.788
     4 SURG   REG   134   1   134   0   7   2   1   1   5   2 1.000

where:

1. U# -- The number associated with the unit.

2. UCBDESC -- A description of the unit (up to eight characters).

3. U_TYPE -- A switch affecting the admission requirements for the unit. This switch setting will not be discussed in this chapter.

4. CAP -- The unit capacity.

5. FC -- The FORCE CRITERION for the unit. The FORCE CRITERIA is the maximum number of days remaining on a patient's current segment of stay that will permit the patient to be considered a CANDIDATE for the FORCE alternate action. The changing of this parameter is not discussed in this chapter.

6. NBCAP -- The NBMAXCAP parameter for the unit (see NBMAXCAP CHANGE subcommand).

7. UA -- The UNIT ALLOWANCE for the unit. The UNIT ALLOWANCE is not discussed in any depth in this chapter though it is briefly mentioned in the BMAXCAP CHANGE subcommand.

8. #CU -- The number of co-units associated with the unit.

9. #AM -- The number of AM emergency streams associated with the unit.

10. #PM -- The number of PM emergency streams associated with the unit.

11. #SC -- The number of schedule/call-in stream pairs associated with the unit.

12. #IP -- The number of input ports associated with the unit.

13. #OP -- The number of output ports associated with the unit. This model component is not discussed in this chapter since the alteration of output ports is not a part of the management engineer's simulation efforts.

14. BBEDS -- This column displays the mean of the BADBEDS distribution associated with the unit (see BADBEDS CHANGE subcommand).

4.   The ASCS-II EXIT Command

Prototype --

     --CMD: EXIT

     The EXIT command is the intended way to terminate execution
of the ASCS-II program and return to MTS command mode. Once the
EXIT command is executed, statistics are printed describing the
program session and reentry to the ASCS-II program can only be
made via the program start-up procedures (see section VIII.G.2.).

Example:

```
--CMD: EXIT
CCID   DATE       TIME      ELAPSED   CPUTIME    COST   PROGRAM      MODEL
-----------------------------------------------------------------------------
WXYZ 11-18-81--16:25:14  00:08:46   1.006731   0.81   ASCS-II        903
<*><*><*>   NORMAL TERMINATION   <*><*><*>
```

where:

     1.   CCID -- The CCID from which ASCS-II was run.

     2.   DATE -- The date that ASCS-II program execution began.

     3.   TIME -- The time of day that ASCS-II program execution
          began.

     4.   ELAPSED -- The elapsed time for the ASCS-II program
          session.

     5.   CPUTIME -- The Central Processing Unit time consumed by
          the ASCS-II program session.

     6.   COST -- The approximate cost of the ASCS-II session.

     7.   PROGRAM -- The program name (ASCS-II).

     8.   MODEL # -- The on-line model number when "EXIT" was
          issued.

     Note, to temporarily suspend ASCS-II program execution and
return to MTS command mode without terminating the session,
simply issue "$MTS" in response to any ASCS-II prompting
messages. When ready to restart ASCS-II, issue "$RES" from MTS
command mode and ASCS-II will resume processing by reissuing the
same prompting message that appeared when program execution was
suspended.

5. The ASCS-II FETCH Command

Prototype --

    --CMD: FETCH

The FETCH command is designed to reconstruct a model on-line
that has been previously constructed and saved in off-line disk
storage. The reconstruction process is carried out entirely by
the ASCS-II program and is transparent to the user.

Example:

    --CMD: FETCH
    P1) ENTER FDNAME (LINE) CONTAINING MODEL: line_file_name
    P2) ENTER FDNAME (SEQ) CONTAINING DISTRIBUTIONS:seq_file_name

    CMD:

In the above example, the first prompting message, after the
FETCH command, requests the name of a "line file" (FDNAME
(LINE)). This file contains the model's structure and many of
the values needed for model initialization. The next prompting
message requests the name of a "sequential file" (FDNAME (SEQ)).
This file contains the distributions that are an integral part of
the simulation model. The counterpart of the FETCH command is
the ASCS-II "SAVE" command in which the same sort of prompting
sequence is encountered to save a model in off-line disk storage.
    If ASCS-II already has a model on-line when the FETCH command
is issued, then the user is informed of the existing model and is
asked whether it should be purged so that another model can be
brought on- line. If the user answers "YES," then ASCS-II purges
the existing model and proceeds with the prompting sequence to
FETCH the new model on-line. If the answer is "NO," then program
control continues with ASCS-II command mode, with the current
model still on-line.

6. The ASCS-II SAVE Command

Prototype --

    --CMD: SAVE

The SAVE command is designed to save the current on-line
model in off-line disk file storage in order that the same model
can be easily reconstructed and brought back on-line at a later
time. The model is saved as is with all of its current parameter
settings and distributions, but all values contained in the
model's statistics collection variables due to simulation are
lost.

Example:

    --CMD: SAVE

    01) ENTER "SAVE MODEL (LINE)" FDNAME: line_file_name
    02) ENTER "SAVE DISTRIBUTION (SEQ)" FDNAME: seq_file_name

    -CMD:

In the above example, the first prompting message, after the
SAVE command, requests the name of a line file ("SAVE MODEL
(LINE)" FDNAME). This file will contain the model's structure
and many of the values needed for model initialization. The next
prompting message requests the name of a sequential file ("SAVE
DISTRIBUTION (SEQ)" FDNAME). This file will contain the
distributions that are an integral part of the simulation model.
During the final stages of the simulation process, the user
performs numerous simulations in pursuit of the final simulation
model. This process may span a number of terminal sessions.
Because of a limited amount of permanent disk space assigned to
the user's CCID, it will become necessary at some point to
$DESTROY some of the intermediate models that have accumulated.
To do so for the latest model saved before the model currently
on-line (which is a later version still) is saved could prove to
be a costly error if the MTS system happens to crash in the
process.   Two methods and examples are presented below to
illustrate safe procedures for saving a current model while
destroying an intermediate model:

    1. From ASCS-II command mode, create new permanent line and
        sequential files by issuing the two commands: "$CRE
        newline" and "$CRE newseq TYPE=SEQ"; where "newline" is
        the name of a new line file and "newseq" is the name of a
        new sequential file.

    2. Save the current model on-line in the files "newline" and
        "newseq".

    3. Destroy the old line and sequential files "oldline" and
        "oldseq" by issuing the $DESTROY commands from ASCS-II
        command mode.

or

    1. Create a new temporary sequential file by issuing from
        ASCS-II command mode: "$CRE -tempseq TYPE=SEQ", where
        "-tempseq" is the name of the new temporary sequential
        file.

    2. Save the model in a new temporary line file (to be
        created implicitly) and the newly created temporary
        sequential file.

3. Issue "$MTS" to suspend ASCS-II execution and go to MTS command mode.

4. $RENAME the temporary files to be permanent files.

5. $DESTROY the old intermediate permanent model files.

6. Restart the ASCS-II program by issuing "$RES."

These two methods are illustrated by the following sequences.

Example #1:

```
 --CMD: $CRE NEWLINE
##CRE NEWLINE                        (this is an MTS echo, not user's input)
# FILE 'NEWLINE' HAS BEEN CREATED.
 --CMD: $CRE NEWSEQ TYPE=SEQ
##CRE NEWSEQ TYPE=SEQ                (this is an MTS echo, not user's input)
# FILE 'NEWSEQ' HAS BEEN CREATED.
 --CMD: SAVE
 01) ENTER 'SAVE MODEL (LINE' FDNAME: NEWLINE

 02) ENTER 'SAVE DISTRIBUTION (SEQ)' FDNAME: NEWSEQ

 --CMD: $DES OLDLINE OK
##DES OLDLINE OK                     (this is an MTS echo, not user's input)
#DONE                                (MTS confirmation)
 --CMD: $DES OLDSEQ OK
##DES OLDSEQ OK                      (this is an MTS echo, not user's input)
#DONE                                (MTS confirmation)
 --CMD:
```

Example #2:

```
 --CMD: $CRE -TEMPSEQ TYPE=SEQ
##CRE -TEMPSEQ TYPE=SEQ              (this is an MTS echo, not user's input)
# FILE '-TEMPSEQ' HAS BEEN CREATED.
 --CMD: SAVE
 01) ENTER 'SAVE MODEL (LINE' FDNAME: -TEMPLINE

 02) ENTER 'SAVE DISTRIBUTION (SEQ)' FDNAME: -TEMPSEQ

 --CMD: $MTS
##RENAME -TEMPLINE NEWLINE
#DONE                                (MTS confirmation)
##RENAME -TEMPSEQ NEWSEQ
#DONE                                (MTS confirmation)
##DES OLDLINE OK
#DONE                                (MTS confirmation)
##DES OLDSEQ OK
#DONE                                (MTS confirmation)
##RES
 --CMD:
```

7.   The ASCS-II SET Command

The ASCS-II SET command is used to set a number of program and model parameters and switches, some of which are simply helpful aids, others of which are essential in the simulation process.   The SET command has a submode so that after the first SET command is issued, ASCS-II will continue to prompt the user from the SET submode.   For this chapter only six SET submode keywords will be described.

a.   The ADJFACT Keyword of the SET Submode.

Prototype --

     SET: ADJFACT { ON | OFF }

The ADJFACT keyword is used to engage (ON) or disengage (OFF) the use of the adjustment factors during simulation.   If a fixed seed has been set and engaged and the model has undergone the adjustment procedure (see section VIII.H.1.), then engaging the ADJFACT switch results in the emergency streams and queue request generators producing the intended numbers of patients and requests for the length of simulation used in the adjustment process.   If the ADJFACT switch is disengaged, then emergency arrivals and queue request rates may differ from the intended rates significantly (in terms of the percent difference of the intended rates: the higher the intended rate, the lower the percent difference).   If the ADJFACT switch is disengaged, then the resulting emergency and request queue arrival rates would be the same as when all adjustment factors are set to 1.0 and the ADJFACT switch is engaged.

Example:

     SET: ADJFACT ON

b.   The AVG&TOT Keyword of the SET Submode.

Prototype --

     SET: AVG&TOT { ON | OFF }

The AVG&TOT keyword is used to choose one of two formats to be used during the production of simulation statistics.
     If the AVG&TOT program switch is engaged (ON), then the output will contain separate columns for weekly totals and daily averages in addition to the day of the week specific statistics for each line of statistics.   For those statistics in which weekly totals have no meaning (percent occupancy, number of beds

occupied, etc), both weekly totals and daily averages will
contain the daily average statistic. If the user has a terminal
capable of printing 132 characters per line or more, then this
switch setting is advised.

If the AVG&TOT switch is not engaged, then the simulation
statistics output will contain only one column in addition to the
day of the week specific statistics for each line of statistics.
This column will contain the weekly totals statistic where
appropriate and the daily averages otherwise. This switch
setting is advised for those users with terminals not capable of
printing 132 characters per line.

Examples:

        SET: AVG&TOT ON

results in the following type of statistics lines being produced
after simulation:

TOTAL	AVG. *	SUN	MON	TUE	WED	THU	FRI	SAT	
379.16	379.16 *	366.01	384.62	388.79	389.43	388.99	376.75	359.51	AVG. #BEDS OCCUPIED
85.01	85.01 *	82.06	86.24	87.17	87.32	87.22	84.47	80.61	AVG. % OCCUPANCY
39.06	5.58 *	4.65	6.70	6.20	5.69	5.18	5.61	5.03	AM EMERGENCY ADMISSIONS
164.20	23.46 *	19.34	28.16	25.44	24.36	23.03	23.12	20.75	PM EMERGENCY ADMISSIONS
203.26	29.04 *	23.99	34.86	31.64	30.05	28.21	28.73	25.78	TOTAL EMERGENCY STATISTICS
49.20	7.03 *	8.12	10.09	9.00	10.00	8.00	2.99	1.00	SCHEDULED ADMISSIONS
24.29	3.47 *	3.57	2.51	2.94	2.78	3.52	5.18	3.79	REGULAR CALLIN ADMISSIONS

whereas --

        SET: AVG&TOT OFF

results in the following type of statistics being produced after
simulation:

TOT&AVG	SUN	MON	TUE	WED	THU	FRI	SAT	
379.16	366.01	384.62	388.79	389.43	388.99	376.75	359.51	AVG. #BEDS OCCUPIED
85.01	82.06	86.24	87.17	87.32	87.22	84.47	80.61	AVG. % OCCUPANCY
39.06	4.65	6.70	6.20	5.69	5.18	5.61	5.03	AM EMERGENCY ADMISSIONS
164.20	19.34	28.16	25.44	24.36	23.03	23.12	20.75	PM EMERGENCY ADMISSIONS
203.26	23.99	34.86	31.64	30.05	28.21	28.73	25.78	TOTAL EMERGENCY STATISTICS
49.20	8.12	10.09	9.00	10.00	8.00	2.99	1.00	SCHEDULED ADMISSIONS
24.29	3.57	2.51	2.94	2.78	3.52	5.18	3.79	REGULAR CALLIN ADMISSIONS

        c.   The FIXSEED Keyword of the SET Submode.

Prototype --

        SET: FIXSEED { ON | OFF } [xxxxxxx]

where: "xxxxxxx" is the desired seed.

The FIXSEED keyword (note, it is not spelled FIXEDSEED) is used to specify a number as the fixed seed and also to engage or disengage the fixed seed process; i.e., the use of the fixed seed as the initial seed to be automatically used at the start of every simulation (see section VIII.G.3.). Because the fixed seed is not a part of the model, it must be set each time the user performs program start-up but only after the model is brought on-line. Once set, however, the user does not need to bother with fixed seeds again until a new one needs to be set or the fixed seed process needs to be turned off.

Any time a number is appended to the end of the FIXSEED subcommand, it becomes the new fixed seed. To be an acceptable seed, the number must be odd and greater than zero.

If the user never engages the fixed seed or turns it OFF after it has been previously engaged, then an initial seed will be picked at random each time the model is simulated. If the user sets the fixed seed value, then any time the fixed seed process is engaged, the same fixed seed value will be used as the initial seed for simulation until the fixed seed process is disengaged or the fixed seed value is changed.

Examples:

        SET: FIXSEED ON 2390785
                .
                .
                .

        SET: FIXSEED OFF
                .
                .
                .

        SET: FIXSEED ON

    d.   The PRINT Keyword of the SET Submode.

Prototype --

        SET: PRINT { ON | OFF } [filename]

The PRINT keyword is used to specify a printfile filename and to engage or disengage the printfile process; i.e., directing output to the printfile instead of the user's terminal that results from the "DISPLAY MODEL" and "XEC" commands. This is a program control device and as such must be set whenever the user wants to make use of this feature.

To set the printfile filename, simply include a legal line filename in the SET PRINT subcommand. The printfile filename specified will remain as such throughout the rest of the ASCS-II session until changed. Output from the "XEC" and "DISPLAY MODEL" commands will be placed at the end of the printfile when the printfile process is engaged (ON) and be printed at the user's terminal when disengaged (OFF).

Examples:

        SET: PRINT ON -AA
                    .
                    .
                    .
        SET: PRINT OFF
                    .
                    .
                    .
        SET: PRINT ON

        e.   The QFORCE Keyword of the SET Submode.

Prototype --

        SET: QFORCE { ON | OFF }

     The QFORCE keyword is used to control the process of FORCED
CALL-INS when a model contains the REQUEST QUEUE component used
with one or more call-in streams.   The QFORCE switch is a model
switch and its setting is therefore saved along with the model.
     If the model utilizes the request queue and the QFORCE model
switch is engaged (ON), then patients will be called into the
model on a FORCED basis when necessary.   If the model utilizes
the request queue and the QFORCE switch is not engaged (OFF),
then patients on the call-in request queue can only enter the
model via the REGULAR call-in process.   If the model hasn't any
request queue components, then the setting of the QFORCE model
switch has no effect.

Example:

        SET: QFORCE ON

        f.   The XHEAD Keyword of the SET Submode.

Prototype --

        SET: XHEAD { ON | OFF }

     The XHEAD keyword is used to control the printing of the
automatic message that occurs when the "XEC" command is issued
(called the XEC HEADER message).   This message conveys
information about the simulation about to be described
statistically; specifically:

     1.   The date and time of day the simulation was performed.

2. The initial seed used in the simulation.

3. The warmup period and the length of simulation (in weeks).

If the XHEAD program switch is engaged (ON), then the XEC HEADER will be printed with every XEC command. If it is disengaged (OFF), then the XEC HEADER message is suppressed. Upon ASCS-II program start-up, XHEAD defaults ON.

Example:

        SET: XHEAD OFF

This would suppress the following type of XEC HEADER messages:

```
****** SIMULATION RESULTS -- 10/26/81 -- 01:41:32 -- SEED = 190358247
        WARMUP = 25 WEEKS  -- LENGTH OF SIMULATION = 200 WEEKS
```

    8.   The ASCS-II SIMULATE Command

Prototype --

    --CMD: SIMULATE # OF WEEKS TO BE SIMULATED

The SIMULATE command is the ASCS-II command to be issued when the user wants to simulate the on-line model with all of its current parameter settings as well as with all of the current program switch and parameter settings. The "# OF WEEKS TO BE SIMULATED" parameter that accompanies the SIMULATE command is the user's specification to ASCS-II of how many weeks the model will be simulated after the model has warmed up (see section VIII.G.4.).

Example:

```
    --CMD: SIMULATE 100
       --   SEED=        190358257
    10/26/81 -- 01:21:01
    <*><*>   SIMULATION COMPLETED  <*><*>

    --CMD:
```

Because the ASCS-II program is also used to build models and change the structure of existing models, a checking routine is used to verify that all of the model's components have been completely initialized prior to simulation. This routine is invoked prior to simulation every time a new model is brought on line via the FETCH command or structural alterations have been made to the current model since the last time the checking routine was invoked. When the model checking routine is invoked, the following message appears after the user issues the SIMULATE command:

WARNING--THIS MODEL IS BEING CHECKED BEFORE SIMULATING

Though the management engineer will encounter this message from time to time, there should never be an occasion in which this checking routine should find a model component uninitialized.

If the user omits the "# OF WEEKS TO SIMULATE" parameter in the SIMULATE command, then ASCS-II will prompt the user with:

Q1) ENTER # OF WEEKS TO SIMULATE:

9.   The ASCS-II XEC Command

Prototype --

     XEC: [F=xecfilename] XEC LINE # RANGE ...

The XEC command is used to produce formatted simulation statistics output based on ASCS-II commands contained in an off-line file called the XECFILE. It is not the intent of this chapter to describe the set up of XECFILEs, only to describe their use once they are setup.

In the prototype, the parameter "F=xecfilename" must be specified only when there has been no previous specification of the XECFILE or the previously specified XECFILE filename needs to be changed.

The "XEC LINE # RANGE" corresponds to the line numbers of the commands contained in the XECFILE and works in the same manner as any other ASCS-II range parameter. The ellipsis marks "..." indicate that there can be any number of line number ranges included in the command as long as they are separated by blanks.

Examples:

     --CMD: XEC F=XFILE ALL
            .
            .
            .

and

     --CMD: XEC 1-25 30-32 75-93 102 106 110
            .
            .
            .

If the "PRINT" switch has been engaged and a PRINTFILE has been specified via the SET command, then all output resulting from the XEC commands is placed in the PRINTFILE.

To determine specific line numbers for the "XEC LINE #
RANGE," the MTS command to $LIST the XECFILE may be issued.
Though the XECFILE contains commands that are not documented in
this chapter, the commands and their associated statistics
descriptions listed should be sufficiently straightforward to
permit the user to identify the line number ranges of the XECFILE
that produce the various sections of the statistical output.

To minimize the number of keystrokes that can be associated
with this command, two or three XECFILEs are usually set up for a
hospital model. One XECFILE is designed to produce a lengthy set
of simulation statistics which is thorough enough to answer most
in-depth questions on model performance. The second XECFILE is
designed with brevity in mind and is intended to produce only
those statistics needed during the numerous simulations of the
heuristic search. Other XECFILEs, if any, might be set up to
focus on various aspects of the model and to be used only after
the simulation process is completed.

I. The ASCS-II Simulation Process

Based on the authors' experience to date, each hospital and
model has its own special flavor: 1) different structure,
capacities, policies, arrival rates, etc., 2) varying sets of
system objectives, 3) varying abilities to cope with the levels
of complexity of the admissions system requirements resulting
from the final model design, etc. This section describes in a
macro fashion the major aspects of the simulation process that
are common to the majority of the models.

To begin, let the following serve as the definition of the
simulation process:

"The simulation process is the performance of a heuristic
search via simulation to determine the set of ASCS allowances,
and in some cases, the model configuration, that best meets
system objectives and constraints."

1. Definition of Simulation Objectives and Constraints

Prior to any simulation, the system objectives and
constraints must be clearly identified. Some of the questions
that need to be answered are as follows:

a. For what hospital services is maximum occupancy a system
    objective?

b. What are the maximum permissible levels for cancellations
    and turnaways for each service and/or blocks of services?

c. If maximum occupancy is the objective for blocks of services, which service(s) shall have their average daily census(es) and admission rate(s) increased to increase overall occupancy?

d. What services are permitted weekend elective admissions and to what extent?

e. What are the desired service specific levels of percent scheduled patients; i.e.,

$$\frac{\# \text{ OF SCHEDULED ADMISSIONS PER WEEK}}{\# \text{ OF SCHEDULED AND CALLIN ADMISSIONS PER WEEK}} \times 100$$

If other factors need to be considered as system objectives or constraints, then they too must be identified.

2. ASCS-II Facts Sheet and Simulation Journal

Once the system objectives and constraints are identified, a facts sheet should be created depicting the major statistical characteristics of the model as they have occurred historically. The facts sheet should also include any of the system objectives and constraints that can be stated quantitatively. Figure VIII-3 represents such a facts sheet.

UNIT NAME	AVERAGE WEEKLY ARRIVAL RATES					AVERAGE LENGTH OF STAY			CONSTRAINTS ON		AVERAGE DAILY CENSUS	BED CAPACITY
	TOTAL	EMERG	URGENT	SCHED	TRANS	TOTAL	EMG&TRN	ELECT	CANCEL	TURNAWAY		
1. ICU/CCU	26.53	17.15			8.38	3.85	3.85			0.17	14.80	18
2. SPECIAL	7.75	0.09			7.66	15.40	15.40			0.00	17.05	16
3. MEDICINE	103.64	78.05	11.59	1.26	11.91	12.10	12.04	12.48	0.01	0.79	179.46	183
4. SURGERY	64.41	28.91	3.22	32.81	1.47	8.81	10.54	7.09	0.32	0.27	78.21	116
5. GYNE	26.34	16.75	0.13	9.38	0.08	4.82	4.22	5.17	0.08	0.15	16.52	27
6. OBS	31.89	29.75		1.94		4.51	4.44	5.68	0.01	0.30	20.43	30
7. LAB&DEL												8
8. PEDS	32.05	27.22	0.19	4.44	0.25	5.17	5.35	4.14	0.04	0.27	23.71	30
9. PSYCH	7.59	7.18	0.18	0.03	0.22	13.83	13.45	20.59	0.00	0.07	14.78	22
10. EMG_RM												10
TOTAL	300.25	204.12	15.28	49.87	30.97	8.55	8.75	7.81	0.50	2.04	367.77	445
TOTAL #2	269.28	204.12	15.28	49.87		8.55	8.75	7.81	0.50	2.04	367.77	427

NOTE: TOTAL #2 EXCLUDES TRANSFERS FROM TOTAL AVERAGE WEEKLY ARRIVAL RATES. IT ALSO EXCLUDES LAB&DEL AND EMG_RM FROM THE TOTAL BED CAPACITY.

Figure VIII-3 Example of a Facts Sheet Used as a Guideline During the Heuristic Search

In addition to the facts sheet, it is important that the management engineer maintain a journal documenting the major simulation models during the simulation efforts. Of particular

interest are the filenames containing the model, the associated
fixed seed and length of simulation for the model, and a
description of the model's major attributes distinguishing it in
the overall simulation efforts. It is not essential to document
every simulation run, but only those representing milestones that
are to be saved on disk file storage. Because of the volume of
paper that the simulation process can produce, the journal can
aid the engineer in systematically plotting and tracking
heuristic search strategy. It will lessen the amount of
duplicative efforts required to ascertain the purpose of
not-so-recent simulation models without referring to old
listings. Finally, the journal provides for continuity from one
resimulation session of the hospital to another. In the event of
personnel turnover, the journal can save a substantial amount of
time, effort, and frustration.

    3. Preparation of the Initial Simulation Model

At this point, it is assumed that from prior simulation
efforts one or more off-line models already exist that are
adjusted for their fixed seeds. It is also assumed that these
models contain the model component structure and length of stay
distributions from which the management engineer can start the
simulation process. Not assumed is that all of the model's
parameter values reflect the hospital's current operations;
however, the correction of any out of date parameter values can
be accomplished by the management engineer.

Because the heuristic search will require numerous
simulations, 100 weeks should be used initially as the length of
simulation in order to minimize simulation costs.

If changes will not be made to the AM or PM emergency arrival
rates, then there is no need at this time to determine a new
fixed seed and reset adjustment factors; simply FETCH an
existing model from off-line disk storage that is adjusted for
its fixed seed and 100-week lengths of simulation. If, however,
the AM or PM emergency arrival rates are to be modified, then
FETCH the most current simulation model, modify the AM, PM and
request queue arrival rates, and perform the adjustment
procedures for a new fixed seed for 100-week simulations.

Once the 100-week simulation model is on-line and the
adjustment for the fixed seed is completed (if needed), make the
necessary modifications to the model's capacities, NBMAXCAPs,
BMAXCAPs, and alternate actions to reflect the hospital's current
configuration and policies. As far as the ASCS-II allowances are
concerned, modify the existing Schedule Allowances (SCHED) as
needed, zero the Cancellation Allowances (CAN), but use the
Census Reduction Allowances (CRA) and the Call-in Maximum
Allowances (CMAX) as they were set when the model was brought
on-line from disk storage. Now SAVE the model; it represents
the starting point in the heuristic search process for the near
optimum schedules.

4. The ASCS-II Allowance Strategies

This section is devoted to definitions and background information for the four ASCS allowances. Guidelines are given to handle the general effects of the allowances, but when nearing the end of a heuristic search, the interaction of the many model variables becomes very subtle; patience in the technique of trial and error is the only advice that can be given. The user must develop his/her expertise through experience and practice.

a. Schedule Allowance (SCHED). From the point of view of the admissions office, the SCHEDULE allowance represents the maximum number of patients for each day of the week that can be given fixed future dates of admission. In terms of the simulator, the SCHEDULE allowance specifies the exact number of patients that will be scheduled for admission on a day of the week basis.

In addition to the administration's objectives, input from the operating room is essential in the setting of the ASCS SCHEDULE allowances. When several individual SCHEDULE allowances need to be set for various surgical specialties, special consideration ought to be given to assigning fixed admission dates to patients with traditionally long surgical procedure times so that their dates of surgery will occur early in the week. In so doing, greater utilization of the O.R. capacity is possible (assuming that this is a consideration).

In general the authors have found, where patients are predominantly scheduled five days per week, that for large units and for sets of units that are co-units of each other, the sum of the SCHEDULE allowances for each day of the week produce good results if their graphical display is similar to that in Figure VIII-4 (this assumes that weekend elective admissions must be kept to a minimum). For Sunday through Thursday, no one day's total schedule should deviate more than 20 percent above or below the mean daily schedule for the five-day period. Note, this scheduling strategy may not be totally feasible in light of the hospital's present needs and/or policies.

The main conclusion to be drawn from the SCHEDULE allowance pattern in Figure VIII-4 is that the early week high admission rates restore the hospital census after, for example, no surgery on weekends. The low end of week schedules result in artificially lower weekend census and as a result have a stabilizing effect on the model's system dynamics.

If the distribution of the sum of the SCHEDULE allowances does not reflect the strategy in Figure VIII-4, it is difficult to predict what effect it will have on the final simulation outcome. It may reduce occupancy significantly (2 percent) or it may not. It more than likely will have an effect on the distribution of call-in admissions across the week. In general the higher the percent scheduled (see the fifth question under VIII.I.1.), the more sensitive the model will be to the SCHEDULE allowances.

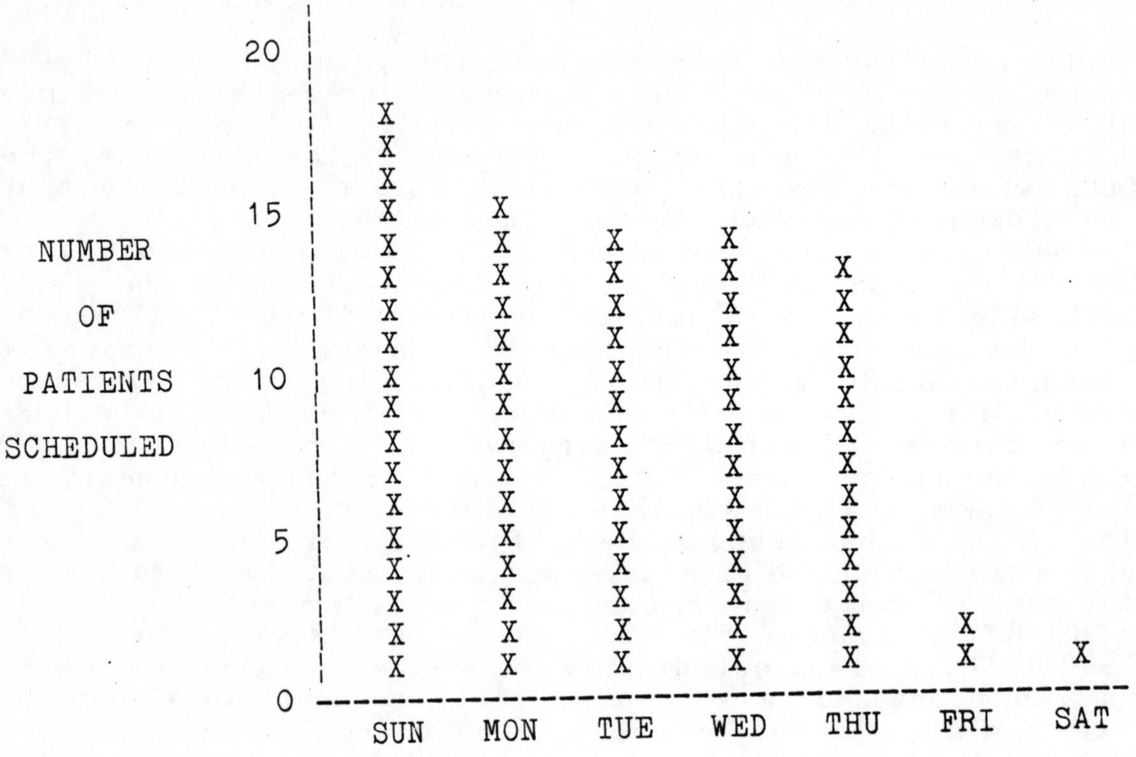

Figure VIII-4 Pattern of SCHEDULE Allowance that has
Historically Produced Good Results

b. Call-in Maximum Allowance (CMAX). This allowance represents the maximum number of patients that can be called in to the hospital on a REGULAR basis (as opposed to a FORCED basis). By restricting the number of patients called in on a daily basis, excessive admissions on any one day of the week are avoided. Thus, undesirably high occupancy situations four or five days later can be avoided when a high demand for empty beds can normally be expected.

Several strategies for the use of the CMAX allowance exist, though the particular strategy for each call-in stream is usually dictated by the unit, model configuration, and CRA strategy used. The first three CMAX strategies listed below assume that there are no request queues associated with the call-in streams.

1) To disable a call-in stream so that no patients will ever be called in, the CMAX should be set to zero.

2) To allow the call-in stream's CRA to be the only controlling factor on the number of patients to be called in, set the CMAX to 99 for each day of the week. This is called the infinite CMAX strategy. With such an approach, it is difficult to tell with certainty how many patients will be called in on any one day of the week even though the average number of call-ins on that day is known over a long period of time. This is due to the fact that the distribution of call-ins for a particular day of the week could be very sparse, covering a wide range of numbers of daily patient call-ins. This approach allows for the quickest recovery of census after holidays and other low census periods. For this reason it is the preferred method for census restoration while keeping cancellations and turnaways in check.

3) This strategy sets the CMAX levels for the weekdays with numbers between 1 and 12 and the weekend CMAXs between a third and two thirds of the average weekday CMAXs. With this strategy it is necessary to consider the volume of call-ins to be attained, the CRA, the distribution of the call-ins across the week and the distribution of the number of patients called in on each day of the week. Given a CMAX of 10 on a Wednesday resulting in .75 simulated call-ins for Wednesdays implies that for most Wednesdays no patients are called in. As a result, raising or lowering the CMAX in this case would probably have little effect on the number of patients called in on Wednesdays. On the other hand, if Wednesday's CMAX had a value of one and .75 simulated call-ins resulted, then 75 percent of the time patients would be called in on Wednesdays. Raising the Wednesday CMAX to four in this model would probably result in about three patients per Wednesday being called in.

4) For those models with request queue generators, the infinite CMAX strategy is normally used. In so doing, the number of REGULAR call-ins is controlled by the CRA but also by the length of the queue; i.e., when the queue length goes to zero, no more patients are available to be called in. If, on the other hand, the queue length never goes to zero, then theoretically the queue length must go to infinity in the limit (assuming that patients are removed from the queue only by the call-in function). As a result, most of the queue's call-ins are admitted on a FORCED call-in basis which significantly reduces the control of the CRA. If a non-infinite CMAX is used with the request queues, then there is an excess of constraints on the REGULAR call-in process which tends to result in increased FORCED call-ins as well as an increased potential for queue failures.

If a service has two call-in streams to a unit, then the first usually uses a low-level CMAX approach (CMAX strategy #2) in conjunction with a low-level CRA. The second call-in stream then uses the infinite CMAX approach in conjunction with a CRA that is the same or higher by as much as 16 than the first stream's CRA for each day of the week. With such a configuration, the first stream has a high probability of bringing in its call-ins every week with regularity (usually the major portion of the total by both streams). The second call-in stream can then restore the census, no matter how low it has dropped, to a safe but suitable level as needed.

For models with a number of call-in streams, usually one unit will have two and the other units will have only one call-in stream each. By assigning the low level CMAX approach to each of the call-in streams, but not to the second in the two call-in stream unit, a degree of equity can be achieved for each of the units regarding the call-in function. If the second call-in stream of the two call-in stream unit uses the infinite CMAX approach and is processed after all other call-in streams, then it can serve as a "catch-all" stream to restore occupancy. As such the "catch-all" call-in stream admits patients regardless of patient service and intended unit of admission.

c. Census Reduction Allowance (CRA). This allowance contains the day of the week specific number of beds to be kept empty following the day's REGULAR call-in process. Its purpose is twofold: 1) It serves to provide a sufficient number of empty beds for emergency admissions throughout the night after all elective patients have been admitted. 2) Due to admission rates normally exceeding discharge rates during the early part of the week, the CRA serves to control the census across the week and thus maintain empty beds for those days when admissions are expected to exceed discharges.

During the heuristic search, the CRA is the primary allowance to undergo modification after modification. In general, if the CRA is raised for one day of the week, then the occupancy for that day is lowered (and vice versa). Once the model's occupancy is up and turnaways are being produced (about one-half percent of the emergency arrival rates), it is hard to predict the exact effect on the occupancy for the other days of the week due to a raise in one day's CRA. The effect on the turnaway rate due to the CRA being raised for one day is usually a reduction in the turnaway rate for that day and also for the next. However, the raising of one day's CRA does not necessarily decrease the week's total rate of turnaways. Similarly, once cancellations occur with sufficient frequency, the CRA will have the same effect on them as it does on the turnaways.

Figure VIII-5 illustrates four hypothetical CRAs for large units or sets of co-units. To say a particular type of CRA is correct would have to depend on the situation as well as the corresponding CMAX allowance used. In general, to obtain an even distribution of call-ins across the week, it is necessary to artificially lower the weekend occupancy through a combination of the SCHED, CMAX and CRA allowances. This in effect promotes bed availability during the weekdays when the scheduled and emergency admission demand is higher and the discharge rates are lower.

Each of the four CRAs in Figure VIII-5 has the potential to yield a uniform number of call-ins across the week given an appropriate setting of the CMAX allowance. For CRA#1 and CRA#2, this requires a low weekend (Friday and Saturday) CMAX allowance relative to the rest of the week. For CRA#3 and CRA#4, a higher weekend CMAX is possible because the CRA itself is more effective in the constraint of weekend call-ins and occupancy.

Because each model is different and the needs and policies vary from one hospital to another, it is not possible to recommend a particular CRA strategy. It is up to the user to determine the CRA or CRAs that best meet the simulation objectives and constraints.

d. Cancellation Allowance (CA). This ASCS allowance is the number of beds to be left empty after processing the stream's scheduled admissions, even if some or all of the stream's scheduled patients have to be cancelled in order to keep the beds empty. The use of this allowance is highly dependent on the hospital's policies governing cancellations. If one of the hospital's objectives is never to cancel a scheduled admission or its ASCS decision rules make no provision for the CA allowance, then the CA allowance should always be set to zero for every day of the week. If the CA allowance is to be a part of the admission system, then the following guidelines are given for its use in the heuristic search:

1) In the beginning, maintain a zero setting for the CA allowance throughout the week while simulating until the number of turnaways and cancellations equals the combined constraint levels for both turnaways and cancellations.

2) Once this combined level is achieved, set the CA allowance so that cancellations occur in the same proportion as turnaways across the week while keeping under the cancellation constraint for the week.

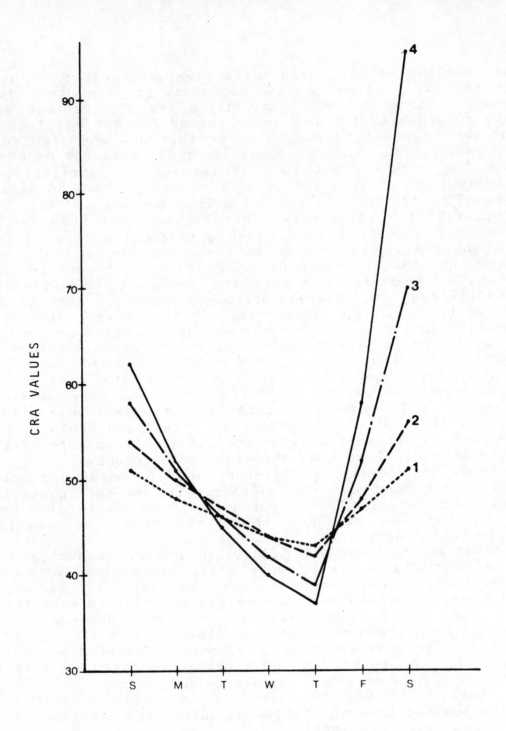

CRA #	:	SUN	MON	TUE	WED	THU	FRI	SAT
1	:	51	48	46	44	43	47	51
2	:	54	50	47	44	42	48	56
3	:	58	51	46	42	39	52	70
4	:	62	52	45	40	37	58	95

Figure VIII-5 Four Types of Census Reduction Allowances (CRA)
Used in Large Units

3) If the number of cancellations is significantly under the cancellation constraint, then the CA allowance levels should be increased.

4) If the number of turnaways is significantly below the turnaway constraint, then attempts should be made to increase the call-in admission rates by adjusting either the CRA(s) or CMAX(s) or both. If request queues are in use, and if the queues are being exhausted, then this is an indication that the call-in request demand is insufficient.

5) If the number of turnaways exceeds its constraint while the cancellation rate is under but near its constraint, then the call-in admission rates should be adjusted accordingly to alleviate the problem.

6) If the combined constraint levels are achieved with the CAN allowance set to zero but the cancellation rate is in excess of the cancellation constraint, then the elective admission rates must be reduced until the the number of cancellations alleviates the problem.

7) If the combined constraint levels are achieved with the CAN allowance set to zero but the cancellation rate is in excess of the cancellation constraint, then the elective admission rates must be reduced until the the number of cancellations is acceptable. This should be a warning signal that excessive admissions on one or more days of the week are compromising the optimal solution. Assuming the emergency rates are properly set, then either the distribution of scheduled admissions or call-in admissions or both are too lopsided. To continue without correcting this condition warrants abandoning the use of the cancellation allowance and obtaining reductions in the elective admission rates and occupancy.

5. The Heuristic Search Strategy

Start the heuristic search using the fixed seed of the initial model and 100-week lengths of simulation. This may involve as many as thirty separate simulations in which the statistics produced are compared to the facts sheet. During this search, it is best to use the abbreviated XECFILE in which only major model statistics are displayed. It is very easy to be inundated by the volume of statistics produced.

Measure each simulation against the facts sheet until the major objectives are roughly met. With each simulation, make minor changes in the CRA and CMAX allowances; the heuristic process is stepwise in nature -- too much change at one time can result in a loss of perspective. Occasionaly, major changes are warranted in the hope that a fresh approach will be more successful. If necessary, minor modifications may be made to SCHEDULE allowances if they have not been rigidly prespecified by administration.

If request queues are incorporated in the model, then the statistics that also should be watched are the queue lengths and the numbers of patients called in according to their queue length of stay. Another important statistic to watch is the number of patients called in on a FORCED basis as opposed to the REGULAR call-in basis. The higher the FORCED statistic is, the more the CRA is being overriden and thus losing its effect. It is desirable to have some FORCED call-ins, but too many with respect to the REGULAR call-ins will compromise the integrity of the call-in process in the eyes of physicians.

If less than maximum feasible occupancy is being achieved and the queue lengths are relatively short, an increase in the request rates to the call-in queues may be in order. By increasing the request rates, it will be possible to call in more patients. This would be done to determine not only maximum occupancy but also how much demand can be placed on the request queues. If this sort of change is made, it is not necessary to perform the adjustment process again for the request queue generators.

In performing the final stages of the heuristic search, methods to restrict turnaways and cancellations are sought. At this point the authors have found that many models are very sensitive to the CRAs for Sunday, Friday, and Saturday. These CRAs also seem to have a high impact on overall model occupancy. The same has also been found to be true for the CMAX allowances.

6. Simulation Model Stability and Fixed Seed Bias

When the heuristic search appears to be over, the model should be saved and, using the expanded XECFILE, a full set of simulation statistics produced.

A verification process attesting to the model's stability and a determination made of the effects due to the use of the particular FIXED SEED is now in order. This process first involves performing the adjustment procedures again to produce two models with the same configuration but using new and different FIXED SEEDS and using 200-week lengths of simulations. If 200-week simulation models adjusted for different fixed seeds and the present AM and PM emergency arrival rates already exist, then they may be brought on-line and modified to reflect the 100-week simulation model in lieu of performing the adjustment process to produce new models. For each of these adjusted models, reset the allowances as they were at the end of the heuristic search and then save them in off-line disk files. Simulate each of these models with their corresponding fixed seeds for 200 weeks. If their simulation output still meets the system objectives and constraints, then all that is left in the simulation process is to: 1) produce the simulation statistical output using the expanded XECFILE, 2) produce a model display (using the DISPLAY MODEL command) for the most representative of the 200-week simulations and 3) document the final model in the journal of simulations.

If one or both of the 200-week simulation models do not meet the objectives and/or constraints, then more heuristic searching is in order. Based on a comparison of the three models' outputs, a determination must be made as to which of the three models reflected the most seed bias. Depending on the determination, several courses of action are possible:

a. A third 200-week simulation model adjusted with a new FIXED SEED can be produced and used in the comparison.

b. A second 100-week simulation model adjusted with a new FIXED SEED can be produced and used in the heuristic search.

c. The heuristic search can be pursued using one of the two (three) 200-week simulation models.

d. The heuristic search can be performed with any of the models with the FIXSEED and ADJFACT switches disengaged (100-week lengths of simulation are used). With this tactic, repetitive simulations using the same allowances reveal the major effects on occupancy and call-in admission rates that can be attributed to the particular sets of allowances. By periodically changing allowances during this process, a stable configuration can be found and used when the FIXSEED and ADJFACT switches are engaged once again and then tested with the 200-week simulation models.

The ultimate test of the final simulation is that two 200 week simulation models, adjusted for different FIXED SEEDS, produce favorable results when using the same allowances.

J.   ASCS-II Simulation Statistics Output

Though XECFILEs are tailored for particular hospital simulation models, the resulting statistical outputs for the majority of hospital models share many common characteristics. Historically, these outputs have featured a section of statistics titled "OVERALL STATISTICS," detailing the model's overall performance, followed by sections for each of the model's units, detailing their individual unit performances. Within each section, lines of statistics are grouped according to the nature of their performance measure. Usually, only those groups of statistics pertinent to a unit are included in the unit's section.

Figure VIII-6 presents two sections of simulation statistics that contain the groups of statistics common to many ASCS-II simulation outputs. For purposes of annotation, the left-most column in Figure VIII-6 contains a line number for each line of the computer printout. This line number column is not part of the normal ASCS-II simulation statistics. The following is the annotation for individual lines of statistics and their groupings:

LINE
NUMBERS   ANNOTATION FOR FIGURE VIII-6
-------   ---

1-2   The XEC HEADER is automatically printed at the start of the output if the "XHEAD" switch is engaged.

6-34   The section of the model titled "OVERALL STATISTICS" describes the model's performance in terms of the entire model.

9-11   Overall hospital census and occupancy.

11   Sometimes it is desirable to know the occupancy for the hospital with the beds from certain units excluded from the calculations.

13-19   The number of admissions throughout the hospital by type of admission.

15   The sum of line 13 and line 14.

19   The sum of line 17 and line 18.

21-22   The totals of the major constraint statistics throughout the hospital; i.e., cancellations and turnaways.

23   DELAYED PATIENT DAYS represents the number of patient days in which patients reside off unit after an attempt(s) to transfer them to a unit(s) that can most satisfactorily care for them fails. Patients residing off service as the result of the CO-UNIT and FORCE alternate actions are not included in this line of statistics. The first day of residence in a unit resulting from the REDIRECTION alternate action is also not included in this statistic; however, any day after the first is included. The other source of DELAYED PATIENT DAYS are those patients whose regular transfer attempt(s) to another unit(s) fails and the patient remains on the unit from which the transfer was attempted.

```
 1   ****** SIMULATION RESULTS -- 11/22/81 -- 17:23:41 -- SEED =    1193252097
 2          WARMUP = 25 WEEKS --   LENGTH OF SIMULATION =100 WEEKS
 3
 4
 5
 6                      <*><*>   OVERALL STATISTICS   <*><*>
 7
 8       TOTAL     AVG.  *    SUN     MON     TUE     WED     THU     FRI     SAT
 9      379.16   379.16 *  366.01  384.62  388.79  389.43  388.99  376.75  359.51 AVG. #BEDS OCCUPIED
10       85.01    85.01 *   82.06   86.24   87.17   87.32   87.22   84.47   80.61 AVG. % OCCUPANCY
11       89.42    89.42 *   86.32   90.71   91.70   91.85   91.74   88.86   84.79 % OCCUP. (EXCLUDING L&D AND ERH ==> CAP=424)
12
13       39.06     5.58 *    4.65    6.70    6.20    5.69    5.18    5.61    5.03 AM EMERGENCY ADMISSIONS
14      164.20    23.46 *   19.34   28.16   25.44   24.36   23.03   23.12   20.75 PM EMERGENCY ADMISSIONS
15      203.26    29.04 *   23.99   34.86   31.64   30.05   28.21   28.73   25.78 TOTAL EMERGENCY STATISTICS
16       49.20     7.03 *    8.12   10.09    9.00   10.00    8.00    2.99    1.00 SCHEDULED ADMISSIONS
17       24.29     3.47 *    3.57    2.51    2.94    2.78    3.52    5.18    3.79 REGULAR CALLIN ADMISSIONS
18        2.35     0.34 *    0.20    0.21    0.46    0.45    0.51    0.24    0.28 FORCED CALLIN ADMISSIONS
19       26.83     3.83 *    3.79    2.77    3.42    3.25    4.04    5.43    4.13 TOTAL CALLIN ADMISSIONS
20
21        0.01     0.00 *    0.00    0.00    0.00    0.00    0.00    0.01    0.00 CANCELLATIONS
22        0.84     0.12 *    0.01    0.06    0.07    0.29    0.35    0.05    0.01 TOTAL TURNAWAYS
23        5.65     0.81 *    0.31    0.59    1.26    1.10    1.39    0.72    0.28 TOTAL AVG. DELAYED PATIENT DAYS
24
25       14.18    14.18 *   14.32   13.92   13.83   14.45   14.31   14.06   14.36 ICC TOTAL CENSUS THROUGHOUT HOSPITAL
26       16.79    16.79 *   16.46   16.93   16.76   16.95   16.97   17.03   16.45 IMC TOTAL CENSUS THROUGHOUT HOSPITAL
27      189.32   189.32 *  184.67  192.58  192.67  191.99  192.27  188.49  182.58 MED TOTAL CENSUS THROUGHOUT HOSPITAL
28       80.44    80.44 *   76.01   82.19   84.51   85.18   84.38   78.73   72.11 SUR TOTAL CENSUS THROUGHOUT HOSPITAL
29       20.31    20.31 *   18.92   19.84   20.64   21.53   21.83   20.41   19.01 GYN TOTAL CENSUS THROUGHOUT HOSPITAL
30       19.80    19.80 *   18.78   19.35   20.76   19.29   19.55   20.78   20.06 OBS TOTAL CENSUS THROUGHOUT HOSPITAL
31        0.00     0.00 *    0.00    0.00    0.00    0.00    0.00    0.00    0.00 L&D TOTAL CENSUS THROUGHOUT HOSPITAL
32       23.99    23.99 *   22.84   25.53   24.95   25.15   24.90   23.15   21.40 PED TOTAL CENSUS THROUGHOUT HOSPITAL
33       14.32    14.32 *   14.01   14.28   14.67   14.89   14.78   14.10   13.54 PSY TOTAL CENSUS THROUGHOUT HOSPITAL
34        0.00     0.00 *    0.00    0.00    0.00    0.00    0.00    0.00    0.00 ERH TOTAL CENSUS THROUGHOUT HOSPITAL
```

Figure VIII-6   ASCS-II Simulation Output with Line Numbers for
Annotation

LINE #

<*><*> UNIT #3: MEDICINE <*><*>
(MED)

LINE #	TOTAL	AVG.	*	SUN	MON	TUE	WED	THU	FRI	SAT	
35											
36											
37											
38	TOTAL	AVG.	*	SUN	MON	TUE	WED	THU	FRI	SAT	
39	136.54	136.54	*	136.01	137.19	136.92	136.93	136.67	136.62	135.44	AVG. #BEDS OCCUPIED
40	94.82	94.82	*	94.45	95.27	95.08	95.09	94.91	94.87	94.06	AVG. % OCCUPANCY
41										1.27	AM EMG & DIRECT ADM. TO MED UNIT
42	8.73	1.25	*	1.44	1.85	1.23	1.06	0.79	1.09	3.34	PM EMG & DIRECT ADM. TO MED UNIT
43	15.83	2.26	*	3.24	1.59	1.71	1.94	1.36	2.65	4.61	TOTAL EMG & DIRECT ADM. TO MED UNIT
44	24.56	3.51	*	4.68	3.44	2.94	3.00	2.15	3.74	0.00	SCHEDULED ADMISSIONS TO MED UNIT
45	2.03	0.29	*	0.14	0.85	0.21	0.77	0.06	0.00	2.02	CALLIN ADMISSIONS TO MED UNIT
46	10.40	1.49	*	2.13	1.09	1.15	1.30	0.99	1.72	1.80	TRANSFER ADM INTO MED UNIT
47	11.55	1.65	*	1.53	1.74	1.58	1.61	1.44	1.85		
48										0.00	PATS ADM BY FORCE
49	0.00	0.00	*	0.00	0.00	0.00	0.00	0.00	0.00	0.27	ADM. OF CANDIDATES FORCED FROM OTHER UNITS
50	1.63	0.23	*	0.18	0.21	0.18	0.21	0.28	0.30	0.04	PATS ADM BY REDIRECTION
51	1.33	0.19	*	0.18	0.34	0.23	0.37	0.12	0.05	4.67	PATS ADM AFTER REDIRECTION OR DELAY ELSEWHERE
52	34.21	4.89	*	0.74	2.10	6.08	7.08	6.36	7.18		
53										1.64	MED AM EMERGENCY ADMISSIONS TO HOSP UNITS
54	13.41	1.92	*	1.57	2.68	2.03	1.82	2.07	1.60	7.12	MED PM EMERGENCY ADMISSIONS TO HOSP UNITS
55	65.26	9.32	*	7.17	11.56	10.46	10.78	9.23	8.94	8.76	TOTAL MED EMERGENCY ADMISSIONS TO HOSP UNITS
56	78.67	11.24	*	8.74	14.24	12.49	12.60	11.30	10.54	0.00	MED SCHEDULED ADMISSIONS TO HOSP UNITS
57	2.00	0.29	*	0.00	1.00	0.00	1.00	0.00	0.00	2.57	REGULAR MED CALLIN ADMISSIONS TO HOSP UNITS
58	16.09	2.30	*	2.45	1.52	2.04	1.76	2.16	3.59	0.21	FORCED MED CALLIN ADMISSIONS TO HOSP UNITS
59	1.64	0.23	*	0.15	0.13	0.30	0.30	0.40	0.15	2.78	TOTAL MED CALLIN ADMISSIONS TO HOSP UNITS
60	17.73	2.53	*	2.60	1.65	2.34	2.06	2.56	3.74		
61										2.52	QUEUE # OF PATIENTS GENERATED
62	17.72	2.53	*	2.35	2.47	2.67	2.71	2.52	2.48	0.00	AVERAGE # OF QUEUE OVER FLOW FAILURES
63	0.00	0.00	*	0.00	0.00	0.00	0.00	0.00	0.00	12.45	AVERAGE # OF QUEUE UNDER FLOW FAILURES
64	66.89	9.56	*	13.87	8.16	6.62	6.13	6.77	12.89	15.23	TOTAL POT. # OF CALLINS GIVEN SUFF. DEMAND
65	84.62	12.09	*	16.47	9.81	8.96	8.19	9.33	16.63	1.13	QUEUE: AVG. OVERALL QUEUE LENGTH
66	1.79	1.79	*	0.89	1.71	2.04	2.69	2.65	1.39		
67										0.00	QUEUE: AVG. LENGTH WITH PATS ON QUEUE 0 DAYS
68	0.00	0.00	*	0.00	0.00	0.00	0.00	0.00	0.00	0.61	QUEUE: AVG. LENGTH WITH PATS ON QUEUE 1 DAYS
69	0.86	0.86	*	0.45	0.98	1.02	1.26	1.18	0.49	0.27	QUEUE: AVG. LENGTH WITH PATS ON QUEUE 2 DAYS
70	0.56	0.56	*	0.31	0.43	0.72	0.80	0.94	0.47	0.25	QUEUE: AVG. LENGTH WITH PATS ON QUEUE 3 DAYS
71	0.37	0.37	*	0.13	0.30	0.30	0.63	0.53	0.43	0.00	QUEUE: AVG. LENGTH WITH PATS ON QUEUE 4 DAYS
72	0.00	0.00	*	0.00	0.00	0.00	0.00	0.00	0.00		
73										1.91	QUEUE: AVG. # OF PATS CALLED IN ON DAY 0
74	11.73	1.68	*	1.90	1.49	1.65	1.45	1.34	1.99	0.22	QUEUE: AVG. # OF PATS CALLED IN ON DAY 1
75	2.06	0.29	*	0.31	0.02	0.26	0.22	0.32	0.71	0.22	QUEUE: AVG. # OF PATS CALLED IN ON DAY 2
76	1.37	0.20	*	0.14	0.01	0.13	0.09	0.27	0.51	0.43	QUEUE: AVG. # OF PATS CALLED IN ON DAY 3
77	2.57	0.37	*	0.25	0.13	0.30	0.30	0.63	0.53	0.00	QUEUE: AVG. # OF PATS CALLED IN ON DAY 4
78	0.00	0.00	*	0.00	0.00	0.00	0.00	0.00	0.00		
79										0.84	TRANSFERS FROM MED UNIT
80	5.36	0.77	*	0.53	0.47	0.83	1.00	0.70	0.99	18.26	DISCHARGES FROM HOSPITAL FROM MED UNIT
81	104.01	14.86	*	10.36	10.24	15.30	16.87	14.20	18.78		
82										0.00	AVG. DELAYED PATIENT DAYS ON MED UNIT
83	0.04	0.01	*	0.02	0.00	0.00	0.00	0.01	0.01	0.00	MED TURNAWAYS
84	0.34	0.05	*	0.00	0.03	0.01	0.14	0.16	0.00	0.00	MED CANCELLATIONS
85	0.00	0.00	*	0.00	0.00	0.00	0.00	0.00	0.00	0.00	MED CALLIN TURNAWAYS
86	0.00	0.00	*	0.00	0.00	0.00	0.00	0.00	0.00		

Figure VIII-6 ASCS-11 Simulation Output with Line Numbers for Annotation (Continued)

```
LINE #
------
87     <*><*><*>  CENSUS BREAKDOWN IN MEDICINE UNIT BY PATIENT SERVICE  <*><*><*>
88
89      TOTAL     AVG.  *    SUN     MON     TUE     WED     THU     FRI     SAT
90       0.11     0.11  *    0.11    0.07    0.07    0.14    0.10    0.10    0.21 ICC IN MED
91       0.14     0.14  *    0.09    0.14    0.12    0.12    0.19    0.25    0.10 IMC IN MED
92     135.42   135.42  *  135.03  136.00  135.82  135.49  135.47  135.56  134.54 MED IN MED
93       0.87     0.87  *    0.78    0.98    0.91    1.18    0.91    0.71    0.59 SUR IN MED
94       0.00     0.00  *    0.00    0.00    0.00    0.00    0.00    0.00    0.00 GYN IN MED
95       0.00     0.00  *    0.00    0.00    0.00    0.00    0.00    0.00    0.00 OBS IN MED
96       0.00     0.00  *    0.00    0.00    0.00    0.00    0.00    0.00    0.00 L&D IN MED
97       0.00     0.00  *    0.00    0.00    0.00    0.00    0.00    0.00    0.00 PED IN MED
98       0.00     0.00  *    0.00    0.00    0.00    0.00    0.00    0.00    0.00 PSY IN MED
99       0.00     0.00  *    0.00    0.00    0.00    0.00    0.00    0.00    0.00 ERH IN MED
```

Figure VIII-6   ASCS-II Simulation Output with Line Numbers for
Annotation (Continued)

25-34   The average daily census (ADC) of patients throughout the hospital on a basis of the units in which they would be residing if no patient were off service. For many simulation outputs, this is a subsection of the OVERALL STATISTICS section and may be found under the subsection title "OVERALL CENSUS BY BEST-UNIT."

35-100   These lines comprise one unit section and describe the model's performance for this unit and its associated model components.

35-36   These lines identify the unit (Medicine) and the abbreviated unit name (MED).

39-40   The MED unit's occupancy and the number of beds occupied in the unit regardless of whether the patients occupying the MED unit beds are on service or off service.

42-47   A breakdown of the admissions to the MED unit by type of admission regardless of whether or not the MED was the intended unit of admission to the hospital. These statistics include patients admitted via the CO-UNIT and REDIRECTION alternate actions.

49-52   The levels of admissions to the MED unit under less than optimal circumstances.

49   The number of admissions to the MED unit for which a candidate patient had to be FORCE transferred (alternate action) to another unit in order to make a bed available for an incoming admission on the MED unit.

50   The number of patients who were candidates and were FORCE transferred (alternate action) out of another unit and into the MED unit.

51   The number of off service patients admitted to the MED unit via the REDIRECTION alternate action after failing to gain admission to their intended unit or a satisfactory co-unit.

52   The number of patients admitted to the MED unit on the day indicated who were denied admission on the day before to the MED unit or one of its co-units. These statistics normally include transfers denied admission previously and first-time admissions to the hospital redirected elsewhere.

54-60   The statistics associated with the MED unit's streams (patients intending admission to MED) that indicate the levels of admissions to the hospital by these streams. These patients may or may not have been admitted to the MED unit.

56   The sum of line 54 and line 55.

60   The sum of line 58 and line 59.

62-78   These lines of statistics appear in the simulation output only if there is a call-in request queue associated with the unit's call-in stream. The statistics are stream/queue specific and have no bearing on where a patient resides once the patient is admitted to the hospital. See section VIII.G.2. for additional information on the call-in process involving queues.

62   The number of patients per day that requested admission to the hospital via the MED unit call-in stream. Note, all patients admitted via the call-in stream, both REGULAR and FORCED call-ins, generated requests to this call-in queue; therefore, this request rate represents the maximum number of patients the call-in stream can admit.

63   The queue overflow failure statistic represents the number of requests that had to be disregarded because the patients remained on the queue (without being called in) longer than the "ABSOLUTE MAXIMUM STAY ON QUEUE" parameter.

64   The queue underflow statistic represents the number of additional patients that could have been called in on a REGULAR basis if the queue length had never gone to zero.

65   The sum of line 60 and line 64.

66   The queue length (number of requests outstanding) after the call-in stream has called in all the patients from the queue for the day that it is going to call in.

68-72   This group of statistics is a breakdown by day of stay on queue (line 66).

68   This line must be zero because if a patient is still
          on the queue on the day of the request after call-in
          processing is complete, then the patient is
          considered to have accumulated one day of stay on the
          queue.

72   For this queue, three days was the maximum intended
          stay on the queue. It would be possible for this
          line to be non-zero given a high enough queue request
          rate;   however, being zero indicates that all
          patients requesting call-in admission were admitted
          within the three-day limit.

74-78   This group of statistics is a breakdown of the day of
          stay on the queue on which they were called in. The
          sum of lines 74 through 78 equals line 60.

80-81   These lines indicate the distribution of the patients
          leaving the unit after completing their segment of
          stay upon transfer or hospital discharge.

81   If the "DISBEST" model switch is engaged (ON), then
          this line of statistics indicates the discharges from
          the hospital of all patients, regardless of
          residence, whose intended unit of residence was the
          MED unit. If the "DISBEST" switch is not engaged
          (OFF), then line 81 indicates the levels of hospital
          discharges for all patients whose last unit of
          residence for their hospital stay was the MED unit
          regardless of the discharged patients' Best Unit
          status.

83   The number of delayed patient days accumulated on the
          MED unit. See the annotation of line 23 for details
          on DELAYED PATIENT DAYS.

84-86   Cancellation and turnaway levels associated with the
          MED unit's hospital arrival streams.

86   The call-in turnaway statistic is an ASCS-II
          statistic to identify an ASCS-II simulation system's
          failure. This line should always be zero.

87-99   This group of statistics indicates the breakdown of
          the average daily census within the MED unit by the
          units in which the patients would be residing if they
          were on their intended units (Best Unit status). The
          title for this subsection often reads "unit CENSUS
          BREAKDOWN BY BEST-UNIT" where "unit" is the unit's
          UNIT name.

K.   References

1. Walter, P. and Hancock, W. "Admission Scheduling and Control
      System Simulator II: Documentation for Developing ASCS
      Simulation Models", currently under revision to replace
      "The Admission Scheduling and Control System: A
      Comprehensive Hospital Admissions Modeling and Simulation
      System II", Bureau of Hospital Administration, University
      of Michigan, Ann Arbor, Michigan, Report No. 77-1, May,
      1977.

2. "Merit Computer Network: User's Memo No. 12", 5115 I.S.T.
      Bldg., 2200 Bonisteel Blvd., Ann Arbor, Michigan 48109,
      Revised 9 June 1980.

3. "MTS, The Michigan Terminal System, Volume 1: The Michigan
      Terminal System," The University of Michigan Computer
      Center, Ann Arbor, Michigan, December, 1979.

CHAPTER IX

EXTENSIONS OF THE ASCS SYSTEM

A.   Introduction

The ASCS system was orginally developed to be part of a
program to use systems technology to reduce and/or contain
hospital costs. The ASCS system was chosen as the first system
to develop because the admission of a patient is the major
administrative act that commits the budgeted resources of the
hospital.   The resources that are committed are the bed and the
associated services contained in the per diem rate and also the
ancillary facilities, and for an important segment of the
patients, the operating rooms.

It could be asserted that the use of the ASCS by itself is a
sub-optimal method of containing costs because it does not
specifically take into account the minimum of the total costs of
the beds, the ancillary services, and when appropriate, the
operating room. The sub-optimal assertion can be defended on the
premise that since the bed is the most expensive aspect of stay,
maximizing average occupancy by utilizing the most appropriate
number of beds is the major contribution to cost containment.
Whether or not this is true has yet to be proven.

The extensions of the use of the ASCS system have been in
two directions: operating room scheduling and the sizing and
scheduling of ancillary services.   Both efforts will be briefly
discussed in the following pages in order to provide the reader
with an idea of the direction of these efforts.

B.   Operating Room Scheduling

1. Systems Problems

From a systems viewpoint the typical operating room system
would appear to have considerable potential for improvement. The
average utilization is approximately 45%(1), and in many cases
substantial overtime costs are being incurred.   This low
utilization appears to be due to the following:

a. Present Scheduling Policies

In many hospitals, O.R. patients are scheduled for the day
that the physician requests, provided O.R. time is available.
Since, in a typical situation, the O.R. time available is greater
than the time the O.R. is being used, the number of O.R. cases
that are scheduled can vary widely on a given day of the week as
well as between the different days of the week.

b. Procedure Estimation Practices

Most hospitals do not have a well developed method of estimating the time it takes to do a procedure. This lack of a well developed system usually leads to underutilization because each procedure has a certain amount of time uncertainty associated with it. This uncertainty, if not quantified, causes the estimated procedure time to be on the high side so that each physician will be able to start his/her procedure at a time agreed to by the scheduler and the physician. Block scheduling of course helps because the surgeon can start the next procedure as soon as the O.R. is cleaned, but there is still the problem of determining when all of the procedures of a given block will be done in order to schedule the beginning of the next block.

c. Reduction of Overtime Policies

A policy which is widely practiced is that a non-emergent procedure cannot begin, for example, after 2 p.m. This policy is an attempt to reduce overtime and it does, but it also contributes to low O.R. utilization because the time that the last procedure can be started will vary from day to day and will be a function of the expected times and variances of the procedures already scheduled as well as the procedure that is about to be scheduled.

d. Equity Between Surgeons' Policies

In order to give each physician an equal chance of access to the O.R. facilities, some hospitals have a first come, first served policy concerning the posting of surgical procedures. This policy helps solve the problem of staff equity but it also causes a problem in responding to the surgeon's request as to when a procedure can begin. If the surgeon does not get a good estimate of start time, then considerable O.R. time may be lost because the surgeon cannot be found when the procedure can proceed.

2. Systems Solutions

a. Reduction in the Variation in O.R. Time Used.

The introduction of the ASCS system greatly reduces the variation in O.R. time used between days of the week and between the same days from week to week because the O.R. elective schedules cannot, without higher approval, exceed the number of beds that are guaranteed for the admission of patients. Also, the bed schedules are established with the intent that all of the schedule allowances will be used. The variation in the number of procedures done on the same day from week to week will be at a minimum. The principal variation remaining will be the variation in procedure times.

In many instances, variation in total procedure times between days can also be reduced by the O.R. scheduler using the following algorithm: Post the shorter procedures on the days where the allocated beds for the day of admission are higher and schedule the longer procedures on the days where the allocated beds are lower. For example, if the allocated beds for admission of surgical elective patients are as follows:

SUN	MON	TUE	WED	THU	FRI	SAT
16	15	13	13	12	0	0

then the O.R. scheduler should attempt to schedule the shorter cases on Monday and Tuesday and the longer cases later in the week on Wednesday, Thursday and Friday. If it is found that this is not possible because of the desire to have, for example, the longer procedure time cases earlier in the week, then the allocated bed schedule could be changed to have the greater number of admissions later in the week.

b. Procedure Estimation Systems

To determine the present quality of the procedure times is relatively easy to do, but the importance cannot be overemphasized. The process requires compiling a list of the estimated procedure times and then to compare them with the actual times taken. Wash-up times may or may not be included, but it is preferable to include them because they are a part of the routine O.R. process. If the procedures are being correctly estimated, then the average difference of the estimated and actual procedure times over a large number of cases would be zero. Figure IX-1 is an example of the analysis.

In this example, the average bias is -4.5 minutes. This means that on the average, the procedures times are being underestimated by 4.5 minutes. Also, procedures 5 and 8 are the two biggest contributors to the bias. Investigations of these procedures should be made to determine what factors were not properly taken into account in estimating the times. Typical situations that occur are that the person supplying the estimate was not the usual person, that the surgeon did multiple procedures without informing the O.R. scheduler of his/her intent to do so, and/or that the procedure was an unusual one so that no past experience could be brought to bear.

The point is that if the reason can be found and that there is a good chance that the procedure time can be more accurately estimated the next time, then the bias in the estimation process will be reduced by this process. For example, suppose that it was found that procedure 8 was underestimated because multiple procedures were involved but the scheduler did not properly take this into account. Then, if we assume that this procedure will be estimated correctly the next time, the average bias will be: (-45+20)/10= -2.5 minutes. In order to get the bias to zero we could ask the O.R. scheduler to estimate first as he/she has done in the past and then to add 2 or 3 minutes to the estimate. Future reviews such as Figure IX-1 should show a decrease in the average bias. The authors have had some experience in using this analysis in a community hospital setting. The average bias using the process described decreased from +20 minutes to +2 minutes within three months.

Procedure	Estimated Time (Mins.)	Actual Time (Mins.)	Difference
1	45	50	− 5
2	60	50	+10
3	75	80	− 5
4	80	70	+10
5	30	45	−15
6	120	130	−10
7	100	95	+ 5
8	55	75	−20
9	75	85	−10
10	60	65	− 5
		Algebraic Total	−45

Average Bias = −45/10 = −4.5 Minutes

Figure IX-1 An Example of The Analysis
of Estimated Procedure Times

c. Variance Estimation

Unfortunately, to do the best possible job of scheduling, we need not only to reduce the average bias to near zero, but also to know the variance of the estimated times. In order to illustrate the use of the variance and the importance of the variance reduction an example will be given.

Figure IX-2 is a compilation of the estimated time for procedure X and the actual time.

Procedure X

Estimated Time (Minutes)	Actual Time (Minutes)	Difference (Minutes)
60	65	− 5
60	75	−15
60	50	+10
60	50	+10
60	60	0
60	60	+ 5
60	65	− 5
60	65	− 5
60	60	0
60	55	+ 5
	Average Difference	0

By using the procedure described in 2.b., we can reduce the average variance to near zero. However, we need to concern ourselves with the variance of the actual times around the estimated times. The variance of the difference in Figure IX-2 is 61.1 minutes squared and the standard deviation is 7.8 minutes.

    d.   Possible Scheduling Practices

      (1) Scheduling Using Mean Procedure Times

For purposes of our example, let us assume that every procedure takes 60 minutes with a standard deviation of 7.8 minutes. What should we tell the surgeon when he calls and asks if a procedure can be scheduled? Assuming the shift starts at 7:00A.M., one schedule would be as follows:

Time	Procedure
7:00 A.M.	1
8:00 A.M.	2
9:00 A.M.	3
10:00 A.M.	4
11:00 A.M.	5
12:00 Noon	6

Suppose that we have already scheduled the first three procedures and we are attempting to schedule procedure 4. If we tell the surgeon 10:00 A.M., what is the likelihood that he/she can start at that time? The probability is .50. Figure IX-3 gives the distribution of times that procedure 4 can start. Please note that the surgeon could start 2.5% of the time as early as 9:33 A.M. and 2.5% of the time as late as 10:27 A.M (assuming the procedure times are normally distributed).

      (2) Scheduling Using the Range of Start Times

If we tell the surgeon 10:00 A.M., then one-half of the time we will be waiting for the surgeon and one-half the time he will be waiting for the last procedure to finish.

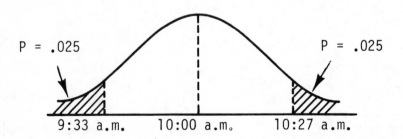

Figure IX-3 The Distribution of Times that Procedure 4 Can Start

The average number of minutes (X) from the beginning of the shift (7:00 A.M.) of Figure IX-3 was obtained by using the following equation.

$$X = \sum_{i=1}^{N} T_i = 3(60) = 180 \text{ Minutes} \tag{1}$$

Where N is the number of procedures that have already been scheduled and Ti is the Average time for the ith procedure.

The range of start times of Figure IX-3 was obtained by using the following equations:

$$ET_{i+1} = \sum_{i=1}^{N} T_i - 2\sqrt{\sum_{i=1}^{N} \sigma_i^2} = 180 - 2\sqrt{(3)\, 7.8^2} = 153 \tag{2}$$

$$LT_{i+1} = \sum_{i=1}^{N} T_i + 2\sqrt{\sum_{i=1}^{N} \sigma_i^2} = 180 + 2\sqrt{(3)\, 7.8^2} = 207 \tag{3}$$

Where:

ET_{i+1} is the earliest beginning time of the procedure from the beginning of the shift.

LT_{i+1} is the latest time that the procedure can start from the beginning of the shift.

σ_i is the standard deviation of the procedure time

With this scheduling approach, we can give the surgeon the range of times and the most likely time. Please note that this scheduling algorithm assumes that each surgeon will begin his/her operation as soon as the O.R. room is available, i.e., no waiting for the surgeon is presumed. We will relax this assumption in a later example.

e. Overtime Considerations

(1) Number of Procedures to Schedule

In B.2.d. how many procedures can be scheduled so that there is a low probability that the O.R. staff will not have to work overtime? If we assume that the O.R. is open for 8 hours or 480 minutes, the answer is determined by:

$$\sum_{i=1}^{N} T_i + 1.645 \sqrt{\sum_{i=1}^{N} \sigma_i^2} \le 480 \qquad (4)$$

Where N is the number of Procedures and 1.645 is the value of the Z transform of the normal distribution that will provide for a probability of .95 that there will be no overtime. Equation (4) is solved by iterating N. For N=7, the left-hand side of the equation equals 454.02 minutes and the average time is 420 minutes.   420/480 x 100 = 87.5 % which would be the expected utilization. Please keep in mind that N for any given day of elective surgery is fixed by the ASCS system.

(2) The Frequency, Range and Average Overtime

In B.2.d. what is the average amount of overtime that the O.R. personnel will have to work, how often will they have to work it and what will be the range?   These questions are posed because we stated the question in section A as a 95% probability that overtime would not be required. Since the average time will be 420 minutes, part of the distribution will extend beyond 480 minutes. Figure IX-4 is a graph of the procedure times.

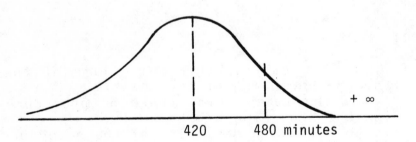

Figure IX-4   The Convoluted Distribution
of Procedure times

(a)   Average amount of overtime that the O.R. personnel will have to work?   Figure IX-5 gives the situation..

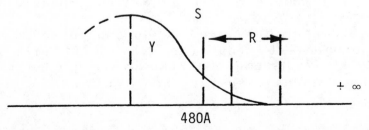

Figure IX-5   The Average Amount of Time O.R. Personnel Will Have
To Work

Figure IX-5   A Part of the normal distribution where A is the mean of the area under the normal curve from 480 to $+\infty$ and R is the Range.

The equation for determining A, the average amount of overtime is:

$$A = \left(Y + \frac{\sigma_p}{\phi(G)\sqrt{2\pi}} \; e^{-\frac{1}{2}\left(\frac{Y-S}{\sigma_p}\right)^2} \right) - S \qquad (5)$$

Where   (G) is the area under the normal curve from S to $+\infty$. (G) is determined by computing y-s/ p and then using a cumulative normal table.

$$\sigma_p = \sqrt{\sum_{i=1}^{N} \sigma_i^2} = 20.68 \qquad (6)$$

For this example,

$$\frac{y - S}{\sigma_p} = \frac{420 - 480}{\sqrt{7 \, (7.8)^2}} = \frac{-60}{20.68} = -2.90 \qquad (7)$$

Thus ϕ (G) $= + .0019$

$$A = \left(420 + \frac{20.68}{.0019\sqrt{2\pi}} \; e^{-1/2(-2.90)^2}\right) - 480 = 4.79 \text{ Minutes} \qquad (8)$$

4.79 minutes is the average overtime that will have to be worked when overtime is required.

In B.2.d. how Often Will the O.R. Personnel Have to Work Overtime?

$$Z = \frac{480 - 420}{\sqrt{7 \, (7.8)^2}} = 2.91 \qquad (9)$$

Where Z is the number of standard deviations between 420 and 480. Using the normal cumulative probability table to find the value of 1-Z, we find that the probability is .0019 of having to work overtime. This means that .19% of the time overtime would be required or once every 526 days.

In B.2.d. what will be the range of overtime that the O.R. personnel will have to work?

To answer this question, we will have to assume that $+\infty$ is 4 in Figure VIII-3. The maximum overtime that would be worked would be: $4.0\sigma - 2.90\sigma = 4(20.68) - 2.90(20.68) = 22.74$ minutes. Thus the range would be from 0 to 22.74 minutes.

f. Scheduling Using Firm Procedure Beginning Times

The problem so far with the examples is that we are unable to give the surgeons a firm time that they can start. The reason, of course, is that each procedure has variability that causes the start time of the procedure to follow to be uncertain. Suppose, however, that we wanted to give the surgeons times that would have a high probability of being the starting times. Using the data from C.2.a. as an example, where all $T_i = 60$ minutes and all $\sigma_i = 7.8$ minutes, we compute the start times by using the following equation:

$$S = \sum_{i=1}^{N-1} (T_i = 1.645\,\sigma_i) \tag{10}$$

where S is the number of minutes from the beginning of the shift to the beginning of the Nth procedure.

Figure VIII-6 contains the starting times.

Procedure	Starting Time Elapsed Minutes	Starting Time Clock Time
1	0	7:00 A.M.
2	73	8:13 A.M.
3	146	9:26 A.M.
4	219	10:39 A.M.
5	291	11:52 A.M.
6	364	1:05 P.M.

Figure VIII-6 The Start Times Where There Is 95% Probability That the Surgeon Can Start At the Time Indicated

Please note that six, not seven procedures can be scheduled as in example B.2.d. If the seventh procedure is scheduled, then it will start at 2:17 P.M. (437 minutes after 7 A.M.) and will not be finished with a high probability before the end of the shift at 3:00 P.M. The O.R. utilization will be 6 x 60/480 x 10 =75% which is a reduction of 12.5% over the 87.5% utilization of example B.2.d. The loss in utilization is because each procedure will, with a very high probability, be finished before the times given to the surgeon for the next procedure to begin.

g. Block Scheduling -- The Determination of the Number of Procedures

Suppose we want to use block scheduling. How many procedures can be scheduled so that there is a high probability that the blocks will not interfere with each other? For example, suppose we have two four hour blocks in an O.R. room for the day. This problem is the same as B.2.d. except that instead of using 480 minutes, 240 minutes or the block size would be used.

3. Discussion of the Assumptions Made In the Systems Solutions

The previous examples are, in a sense, misleading because we have assumed the following:

a. all procedures have the same mean and variance,
b. the means and variances of the procedures are known, and
c. the distribution of procedure times are normally distributed.

Assumption a., that all procedures have the same means and variances, is of course not true. This assumption was made in order to save space in presenting the examples. The equations given are correct when the assumption is not used. However, it is not practical when the means and variances do differ for each procedure's start time to be calculated in advance. What will be needed is a mini or micro computer that the O.R. scheduler can use to determine in real time the start time or the start time range as he/she is talking to the surgeon. The average procedure times and variances would have to be stored on file so that they could be quickly retrieved to be used in the scheduling process.
Assumption b. is only partially true because it is unreasonable to expect that one can collect enough information to obtain the means and variances for all surgical procedures. The computer-aided system has to be designed so that estimates of surgical means and variances can be obtained and inputted from whatever source is most appropriate. An experienced O.R. scheduler will be able to supply good estimates of mean times especially after the procedure as outlined in 2.b. of this chapter has been implemented. The scheduler can use the computer-aided data base to affirm his/her estimates and to supply estimates where the scheduler has no experience. The scheduler will have trouble estimating variances because this has not been required before and it does not have the intuitive content that the average does. One solution would be that the computer would supply the variance by using the coefficient of variation determined from those procedures where the means and variances are known.

Assuming c., that the distribution of procedure times are normally distributed, is necessary in order to use analytic expressions. Little or no data are available to ascertain the validity of the normality assumption. However, the normality assumption is reasonably robust. Even if the distribution of procedure times is not normal, the convolution of procedure times becomes normally distributed with even two or three convolutions. This means that the determination of the number of procedures that can be done on a shift with stated probabilities of overtime, and estimates of starting times, particularly later in the day are good estimates. The problems that may arise would be for the estimates of the procedure times early in the shift. If this becomes a problem, correction factors can be established as a function of the number of procedures.

Another method would be to store a number of points of the cumulative distribution for each procedure where there are sufficient data. The computer could then convolute the distributions in real time when estimates of procedure starting times are needed. For example, if ten points were stored for each cumulative distribution where the points were selected to closely map the right-hand tail of the convoluted distribution could be obtained without requiring abnormal amounts of computer storage.

4. Summary

It is hoped that the foregoing discussion provides the reader with examples of the types of O.R. problems that have an excellent chance of being solved once the ASCS system is installed. Most of the algorithms presented will provide better operational control of operating rooms than presently exists. The use of the ASCS greatly reduces the variation in the number of procedures done each day. This reduction inceases the potential for increased utilization of the O.R. facilities. Increased utilization means that the number of O.R. rooms needed can be reduced, if the demand stays the same, with much better information given to physicians and administration.

C. Ancillary Facilities Planning

1. Introduction

The ASCS can be viewed as a patient flow monitoring process. The ancillary services supply services to the patients as requested by the physicians and other medical authorities. One of the possible extensions of the ASCS is to use it as a vehicle to predict ancillary load demands. Once the demands are known, ancillary facility sizing and staffing can then be best accomplished.

The first attempt to do this is reported in reference (2). The hospital was interested in determining if patient flow patterns (primarily admission rates) could be altered to smooth the workload in the ancillary departments. The ancillary load was due not only to patient flow, but also to outpatient demand.

Thus loads from inpatients and outpatients were predicted separately and then the loads were added to obtain the best picture of ancillary service demand. Both demands were projected to the planning year of the new facility -- 1990. This posed technical problems because the length of stay for the base year of 1976 to 1990 was projected to decrease substantially. Since ancillary inpatient loads for many inpatients are a function of the day of stay and since length of stay reductions tend to intensify the rate of ancillary service required, computer algorithms had to be developed to reflect these forecast changes.

Forecasts of the ancillary demand in 1990 were made for each of the 19 major ancillary departments. Space does not permit a detailed presentation and explanation of the effort, but examples using selected ancillary services as well as general analysis will give an indication of the potential of this type of planning effort.

2. Methodology

The procedure that was used is as follows:

a. The patient flow data of the hospital were obtained for the 1976 calendar year.

b. The data were modified to reflect length of stay reductions and ancillary service intensification and patient arrival rates for the year 1990.

c. Investigations were performed to determine the factors which affect ancillary load. The variables were:

   1) The day of the stay of the patient
   2) How the patient was admitted-elective, urgent or emergent.
   3) The clinical service to which the patient was admitted.

d. The inpatient and outpatient admission policies were discussed with the hospital administration. A range of possible policies was determined.

e. The ASCS simulator was used to simulate the range of policies in order to determine their effect upon ancillary loads. The measure of load used was any procedure that had a billing code.

f. The simulation output representing the inpatient ancillary loads that reflected the admissions policies was combined with the outpatient ancillary loads and presented in graphical form.

g. Conclusions were drawn concerning the most appropriate staffing policies with respect to staffing costs and service requirements.

3. Examples of the Results

   a. Average Use Rates

   Figure IX-7 is a graph of the average number of procedures per day of inpatient stay for all ancillary departments and all inpatients. This figure is presented because it illustrates the general impact of admission on ancillary load. Also, it

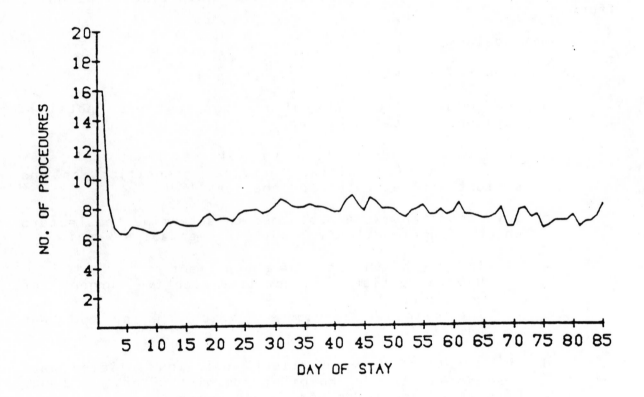

Figure IX-7 Average Number of Procedures per Day of Stay for All Ancillary Departments and All Patients

illustrates the "steady state" load that occurs after the admission activity. This load has a substantial impact on weekend staffing because of the presence of many of the patients in the hospital throughout the weekend period. Also, please note the slight increase in average number of procedures between 15 and 60 days. This is probably because the patients who stay for longer periods required more ancillary services on the average than the vast majority of patients who stayed fewer than 15 days.

b. Admissions Dependency

Of the 19 ancillary services, 14 reflected a substantial increase in demand on the first few days of stay as compared to the remainder of the stay. Thus the day of admission would appear to have a substantial impact on many of the ancillary services (see Figure IX-8).

c. ASCS Simulations of Inpatient Flows

Figure IX-9 is a scenario of the inpatient runs using the ASCS system. Each run is designed to reflect a possible admission policy. The scenarios are somewhat complicated by the fact that two bed capacities are involved: 739 and 660 beds. The first, 739, is the number of beds the hospital was planning to build, and 660 beds is the minimum number that would be needed to care for the forecasted number and types of patients. Because the hospital planners were planning to build 739 beds, the expected occupancy would be less than the maximum average conditions. Since the hospital is planning to operate at less than maximum occupancy, there is a certain amount of latitude regarding when patients can be admitted. This latitude has been reflected in the "simulation objective" column. For example, simulation run #7 is an attempt to smooth admissions Monday through Thursday. The idea is to attempt to smooth the load on the ancillary services for the period Monday through Friday.

The number of days that surgery is to be scheduled is also investigated as well as whether or not urgent admissions can be admitted on the weekends.

Simulation Run #0 is of interest because it is a reflection of the present operating policies of the hospital concerning inpatient admissions and patient flows. It is included so that the hospital executives can compare the results of the present practices with the various alternatives.

Figure IX-10 is a plot of the average number of inpatient admissions vs. the day of week. The numbers refer to the simulation run numbers of Figure IX-9. Please note the following:

(1) Run #0 -- the present operation has declining admissions from Monday to Saturday.

Ancillary Service	Approximate ratio of first or second day procedure rate to the average of the following 18 days of stay.
Heart Station-EKG	10.0
Bacteriology/Microbiology Lab	2.4
Biochemistry Lab	2.3
Immunology Lab	7.5
Lab Test Panel	59.0
Hematology Lab	13.0
Pathology Lab	4.5
Ligand Assay Lab	2.0
SMI Coagulation Lab	4.8
Pediatrics Lab	3.3
Nuclear Medicine	4.9
Radiology – Main	4.8
Radiology – Other	5.3
Blood Bank	4.4

Figure IX-8 A Comparison of the Average Procedure Rate During the First Few Days of Stay as Compared to the Steady State Rate

SIMULATION RUN	CAPACITY	SIMULATION OBJECTIVE	DAYS SCHED. MED, SURG & PEDS	WEEKEND CALLINS
0	NON-SIMULATED DATA SET FROM PROJECTED DATA FOR 1990			
1 (A)	739 (B)	MAX. OCC.	5 (D)	
2	739	SMOOTH ADM. SUN - THUR	5	
3	739	SMOOTH ADM. SUN - SAT	6 (E)	YES
4	660 (C)	MAX. OCC.	5	
5	739	MAX. OCC.	5	YES
6	660	MAX. OCC.	5	YES
7	739	SMOOTH ADM. MON - THUR	5 (F)	YES
8	739	SMOOTH ADM. SUN - THUR	5	YES

A. SETS 1 THROUGH 8 REPRESENT SIMULATED DATA.

	MED	SURG	GYN	BURN	PEDS	M/S SWING	TOTAL

B. CAPACITIES USED BASED ON DATA & OCCUPANCY FIGURES FROM PLANNING OFFICE WHERE ADC FOR PEDS=143.65.

MED	SURG	GYN	BURN	PEDS	M/S SWING	TOTAL
224	250	40	29	192	4	739

C. MINIMUM CAPACITIES NEEDED TO SATISFY PATIENT DEMAND WHERE PEDS ADC=143.65.

MED	SURG	GYN	BURN	PEDS	M/S SWING	TOTAL
205	232	40	29	150	4	660

D. FIVE-DAY SCHEDULED ADMISSIONS: SUNDAY THROUGH THURSDAY.

E. SIX-DAY SCHEDULED ADMISSIONS: SUNDAY THROUGH FRIDAY.

F. FIVE-DAY SCHEDULED ADMISSIONS: SUNDAY THROUGH FRIDAY; HOWEVER SUNDAY'S SCHEDULE RATE WAS SET AT APPROXIMATELY 1/3 THE DAILY RATE FOR MONDAY THROUGH THURSDAY.

Figure IX-9 A Scenario of the Inpatient Runs

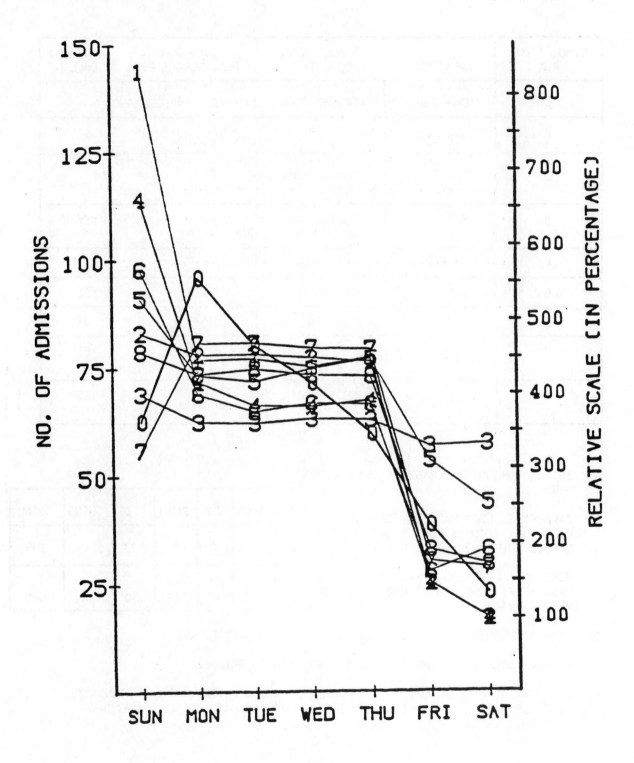

Figure IX-10   Average Number of Inpatient Admissions vs.
Day of Week

(2) The lines from Monday to Thursday (excepting run #0) appear to have approximately a zero slope. This should stabilize the ancillary loads for these days.

(3) The admissions rate on Sunday shows high variability between runs. The highest number of admissions on Sunday is run #1 where maximum average occupancy is desired with no weekend call-ins. Run #5 on the other hand has the same conditions as #1 but call-ins are permitted on the weekend. Sunday admissions are much less.

(4) Run #0, the present hospital practice, indicates low Sunday admissions, but high Monday admissions. The most likely reason for this situation is the desire to keep the ancillary loads low on the weekends.

Figure IX-11 is a series of plots of the overall inpatient ancillary activity load. If the objective is to smooth average actual ancillary load, then:

(1) Runs #5 and #6, which are maximum occupancy runs with weekend call-ins, produce uniform ancillary loads for the period Sunday through Thursday.

(2) The "Smooth Admissions" runs generally produce increasing ancillary loads from Sunday through Thursday. They do not produce a smooth demand as hypothesized. The reasons are that the load for the large majority of the ancillary departments is higher for the first few days of stay, not just the first day. That produces a cumulative load effect.

(3) Run #0, results in relatively low loads on weekends and reasonably level loads for Monday to Thursday. Sunday, Friday, and Saturday have relatively low loads.

(4) If it is desired to have a stable load for the ancillary departments for a five day/week period, then the best five days would be Sunday through Thursday. Runs #3, #5, and #6 accomplish this. Further, the full staffing would enable the O.R. facilities to be used as well on Sunday as for the period Monday through Friday.

(5) Ancillary staffing on Sunday would have to be much higher than the rest of the week for Run #1. This is because Run #1 is for maximum occupancy and does not permit weekend call-ins. In order to restore occupancy, a large number of admissions

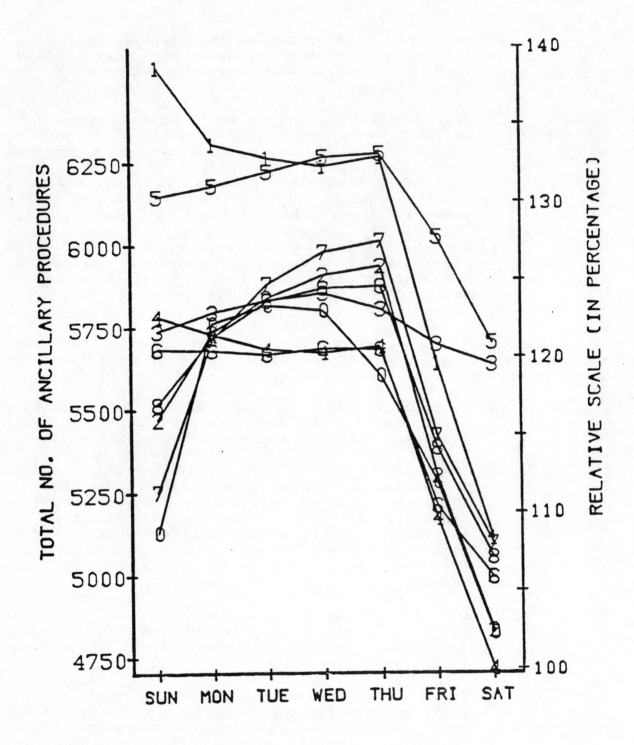

Figure IX-11 Overall Average Total Ancillary Activity –
Inpatient vs. Day of Week

have to be made on Sunday. These admissions require the availability of ancillary staff or the necessary services will not be provided.

d. Outpatient Loads

Figure IX-12 is an example of curves that give the projected number of average outpatient procedures as a function of the day of the week for the laboratories indicated. In each case, the procedures are fairly uniform from Monday to Friday with a slightly higher load on Monday and Tuesday. These curves are a reflection of present practice modified for projected increases in outpatient load for 1990. The curves, of course, can be changed by changing the number of staff and/or hours that the outpatient departments are open. The decision was made that the outpatient demand patterns would not be changed.

e. An Example of the Loads on Bacteriology/Microbiology Laboratories

Figure IX-13 is a family of curves reflecting the load on the Bacteriology/Microbiology Lab due to inpatients only. Figure IX-14 is a plot of the average number of procedures by day of stay by inpatients for the Bacteriology/Microbiology Lab. The activity of this lab reflects a higher demand during the first few days of stay. Figure IX-15 is the total of the inpatient and the outpatient loads of the Lab. The curves appear to be much closer together than those of the inpatient load only (Figure IX-13). This is an illusion due to a change in scale. The conclusions that can be drawn for figure IX-15 are:

(1) Maximum occupancy runs at the 739-bed level (runs #1 and #5) produce the most constant load for the period Monday through Friday.

(2) All of the runs are superior to run #0 with respect to smoothness for the period Monday through Friday. This means that it would be relatively easy to improve on the present operation.

(3) The right side of Figure IX-15 gives a relative scale with 100 being the lowest data point on the scale. If we assume that staff is related to the number of procedures that have to be done, then we can determine the staff necessary on the weekends to provide the required services. For example, if the objective is to minimize the staff required on Saturday and Sunday, run #0 would appear to be desirable because the weekend staff would be projected to be 100/135 x 100 = 74% of the staff during the week. This projection assumes that the work gets done when ordered and that the work is ordered when it should be.

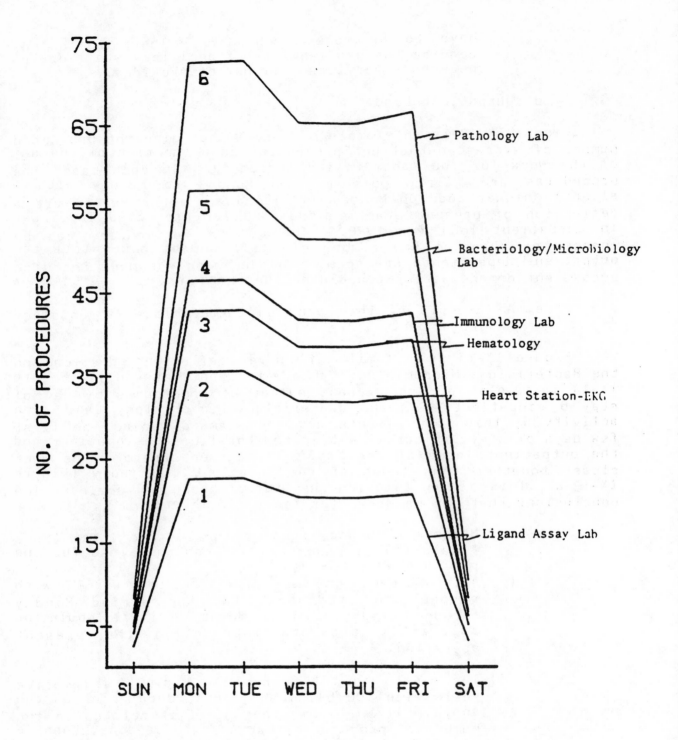

Figure IX-12 Projected Average Number of Procedures Caused by Outpatient Activity in 1990 for Pathology, Lab, Bacteriology/ Microbiology Lab, Immunology Lab, Hermatology, Heart Station-EKG, and Ligand Assay Lab

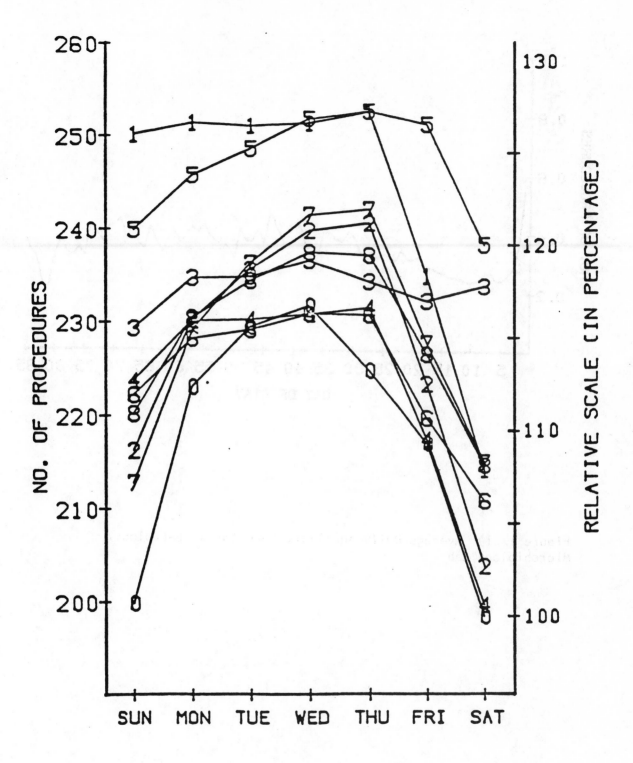

Figure IX-13 Average Number of Inpatient Procedures vs.
Day of Week for Bacteriology/Microbiology Lab

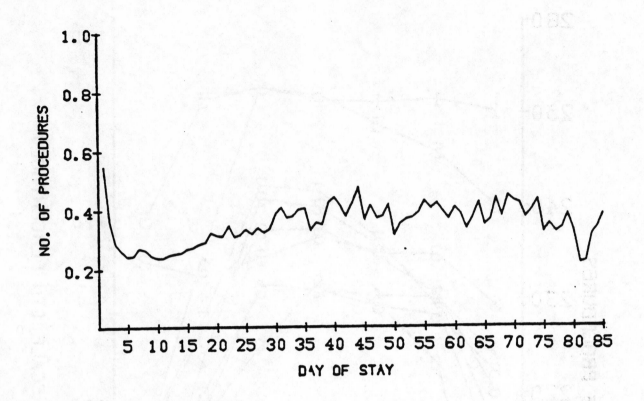

Figure IX-14 Average Daily Ancillary Load for Bacteriology/
Microbiology Lab

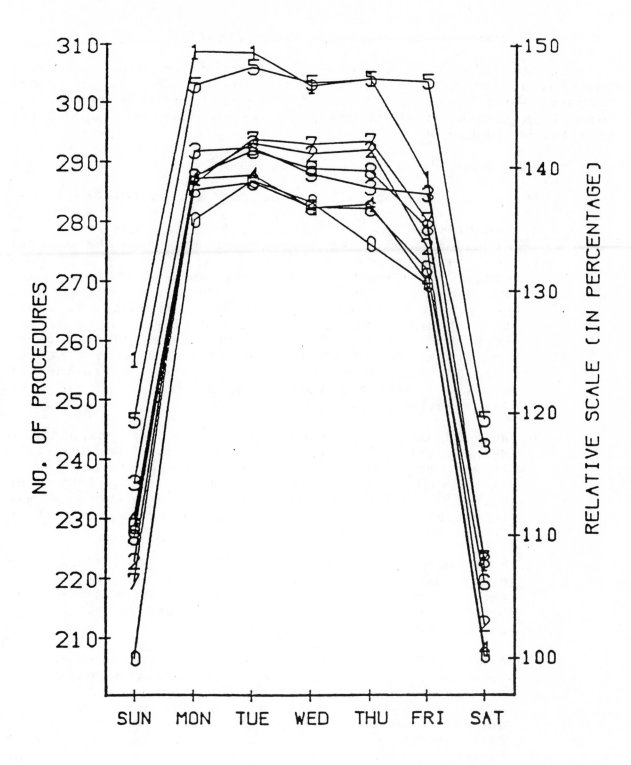

Figure IX-15 Total Average Number of Procedures (Inpatient plus Outpatient) for Bacteriology/Microbiology Lab

f. Summaries of Projected Weekend Loads

Figure IX-16 is a summary of projected weekend loads as a function of the midpoint load for the periods Monday to Friday for simulation runs #5, #7, and #8. These runs were chosen for comparison because they appeared to be the closest to how the hospital would operate.

4. Main Conclusions of the Work To Date

The main conclusions from this work are as follows:

a. Inpatient Patient Admissions Policies do affect the stability of loads on ancillary departments -- especially those departments experiencing a higher demand in the first few days of admission. The variation in load due to the admissions policies is sufficient to affect substantially the number of staff that should be available on the different days of the week. By varying the inpatient admissions policies, ancillary staff loads between days of the week can be reduced, thus enabling the institution to provide the ancillary services with fewer personnel and/or with less overtime.

b. Weekend demand is surprisingly high as compared to demand during the week (70-80% for most laboratories). If we compare the ratio of present weekend staffing in the hospital to the level of staff during the week with the ratios predicted, we can infer that we are incurring excess costs or that the work is not getting done when it should be done.

c. Weekend demand varies widely between ancillary departments. This means that proper staffing on the weekend has to be established on a lab-by-lab basis. No blanket policies about weekend staffing can be made and defended.

d. A hospital that plans to operate at less than maximum occupancy, must consider the maximum occupancy situation so that the extremes in demand can be planned for in terms of space, personnel, and equipment for the ancillary departments. The need to size ancillary units as if maximum occupancy would occur is one of the sources of excess costs of operating at less than maximum occupancy.

e. If we desire to operate hospitals at minimum cost, there seems to be a basic inconsistency between this objective and having the majority of the employees work five days/week -- Monday through Friday. This is because of the serial aspects of patient care. For example, patients have to be admitted on Sunday in

LAB	RUN 5			RUN 7			RUN 8		
	LOAD RANGE MON-FRI	SUN LOAD (AS A % OF RANGE MIDPOINT)	SAT LOAD (AS A % OF RANGE MIDPOINT)	LOAD RANGE MON-FRI	SUN LOAD (AS A % OF RANGE MIDPOINT)	SAT LOAD (AS A % OF RANGE MIDPOINT)	LOAD RANGE MON-FRI	SUN LOAD (AS A % OF RANGE MIDPOINT)	SAT LOAD (AS A % OF RANGE MIDPOINT)
LIGAND ASSAY	52-55	65	62	48-54	57	57	48-53	61	61
RESPIRATORY THERAPY - MAIN	511-515	99	98	489-501	97	98	488-496	97	97
RESPIRATORY THERAPY - MOTT	89-91	97	97	73-78	94	97	74-77	94	97
PHYSICAL THERAPY	233-245	80	80	222-228	79	79	219-227	78	78
PHARMACY	1010-1050	74	73	960-980	71	72	950-970	72	72
HEART STATION	94-106	85	64	82-110	68	56	82-110	80	57
BACTI/MICRO	302-305	82	82	280-293	72	74	278-292	80	78
BIOCHEMISTRY	3090-3140	92	88	2790-2900	84	84	2780-2960	87	83
IMMUNOLOGY	86-90	55	50	76-88	46	45	76-87	47	42
LAB TEST PANEL	140-165	52	34	130-172	38	26	130-168	48	27
HEMATOLOGY	103-124	90	60	89-128	66	49	90-124	83	50
PATHOLOGY	136-153	51	48	134-145	43	44	132-144	45	44
SMI COAGULATION	252-272	97	85	225-275	82	78	225-265	93	79
PEDIATRICS	214-222	70	69	175-193	59	60	173-191	64	60
NUCLEAR MEDICINE	70-76	47	44	65-74	39	39	66-74	44	39
HEMODIALYSIS	3.3-3.6	35	36	3.2-3.5	34	36	3.2-3.5	34	36
RADIOLOGY - MAIN	450-490	56	50	430-490	48	46	430-480	53	46
RADIOLOGY - MOTT	119-125	67	61	97-112	54	54	96-110	62	53
BLOOD-BANK	510-584	104	83	475-575	88	76	470-560	97	78
OVERALL TOTAL (AVERAGE) ANCILLARY ACTIVITY	7450-7800	83	78	6850-7450	76	74	6800-7400	80	74

Figure IX-16   A Summary of Average Ancillary (Inpatient Plus Outpatient) Load for Simulation Runs 5, 7, and 8

order to have surgery on a Monday. Thus if we assume that the O.R. rooms are to be open Monday through Friday, then most of the ancillary services should be staffed by their full-time personnel from Sunday through Thursday. The need for this phase shift is even more evident if no elective patients are permitted to be admitted on Friday and Saturday because, in order to restore the occupancy, many of the patients not admitted on Friday and Saturday have to be admitted on Sunday.

5. Further Extensions

From this work, it is clear that ancillary loads by department can be forecast on a day of the week basis. Further, the workload of this work was done on a computer, the forecasts can be easily refined with the only major limitation being the data base(s) available. Also, the cost trade-offs of staffing at levels more consistent with the demand, with the attendant reductions in length of stay, can also be done on a computer at relatively little cost. The potential of minimizing cost of the patient care by more appropriate ancillary staffing would appear at this point to be very high, especially for the larger hospitals which tend to have a greater number of ancillary facilities.

As an example of the improvements that could be made in the methodology, the following is presented as a method of refining the use of procedures as a measure of load.

a. Determining Staff Required Using Number of Procedures

This present approach assumes that at the macro level, the time and equipment use per procedure will be constant. This is probably a good assumption as long as the procedure mix and the procedure methods do not change. The average staff necessary in each lab on a daily basis can be determined as follows:

(1) Determining the Time per Procedure

A suggested approach is to select days where the people in a lab are known to have a full workload. The time per procedure can then be computed. It is important to use at least 20 days of data in order for the procedure mix to stabilize.

(2) Determining the Average Staff Required

$$AS = \frac{APD \times TP}{WT} \tag{11}$$

Where:

AS = Average staff needed for a given day of the week

APD = Average number of procedures forecast for a particular day of the week.

TP = Time/procedure in hours

WT = Working Time of a staff member/day in hours

There are, of course, more sophisticated methods of determining the appropriate staff. A more detailed analysis could be done by:

(a) Determining the fixed and variable time per procedure or

(b) If the lab has an RVU (relative value unit) system, use the system to determine the time per procedure with any adjustments for forecast mix changes.

D.   References

1. Magerlein, J. Surgical Scheduling and Admissions Control, Report 78-6, School of Public Health, , The University of Michigan, Nov. 1978 (Ph.d. Dissertation).

2. Hancock, W. and Walter, P. "University Hospital Ancillary Services Project" Report 80-1, Management Information Systems Group of the Department of Hospital Administration. Jan. 1980.

3. Hancock, W.; Johnston C.; Magerlein, D.; Martin J.; and Walter, P. "Replacement Bed Size for University Hospital: Determination and Final Results ". Report No. 78-1, Department of Hospital Administration, University of Michigan, May 1978.